HANDBOOK OF
Pediatric
Physical
Therapy

SECOND EDITION

TOBY M. LONG, PhD, PT
Associate Professor
Georgetown University
Department of Pediatrics
Associate Director for Training
Georgetown University Child Development Center
Director
Division of Physical Therapy
Georgetown University Child Development Center
Washington, DC

KATHLEEN TOSCANO, MHS, PT, PCS
Shady Grove Adventist Hospital
Rockville, MD

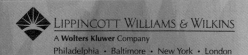

LIPPINCOTT WILLIAMS & WILKINS
A **Wolters Kluwer** Company
Philadelphia · Baltimore · New York · London
Buenos Aires · Hong Kong · Sydney · Tokyo

Publisher: Susan Katz
Managing Editor: Ulita Lushnycky
Marketing Manager: Debby Hartman
Production Editor: Paula C. Williams
Compositor: Peirce Graphic Services, Inc.
Printer: R.R. Donnelley & Sons Company

Printed in the United States of America

Library of Congress Cataloging-in-Publication Data

Long, Toby M.
 Handbook of pediatric physical therapy / Toby M. Long, Kathy Toscano.—2nd ed.
  p. ; cm.
 Includes bibliographical references and index.
 ISBN 0-7817-2799-5
  1. Physical therapy for children—Handbooks, manuals, etc. I. Toscano, Kathy.
 II. Title.
  [DNLM: 1. Physical Therapy—Child—Handbooks. 2. Physical Therapy—Infant—Handbooks. 3. Developmental Disabilities—therapy—Handbooks. WB 39 L849h 2001]
 RJ53.P5 L66 2001
 615.8'2'083—dc21

                                                          2001029688

 The publishers have made every effort to trace the copyright holders for borrowed material. If they have inadvertently overlooked any, they will be pleased to make the necessary arrangements at the first opportunity.
 To purchase additional copies of this book call our customer service department at **(800) 638-3030** or fax orders to **(301) 824-7390**. International customers should call **(301) 714-2324**.

To our families
Bill and Charlie Cox
Attilio, Kristina, and Domenico Toscano

Preface

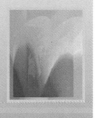

Pediatric physical therapy is truly a specialty area. Children are special people who require sensitivity, understanding, compassion, and patience from adults who guide them in becoming happy, productive citizens. Children with disabilities require the same compassion, patience, understanding, and sensitivity to realize their potential. However, they also need service providers who confidently provide therapeutic interventions in natural environments, who collaborate with family members and other service providers, and who document service provision in a timely manner for a variety of service delivery systems. The children served by pediatric physical therapists often have complex conditions that change over time, requiring constant reshaping of treatment strategies and realigning of outcomes and goals.

The *Handbook of Pediatric Physical Therapy* is designed to provide essential information regarding pediatric physical therapy. It is a succinct resource for therapists needing key information regarding intervention, service delivery, or a particular condition. The *Handbook* was designed to provide information quickly to help answer clinical questions. There are many comprehensive textbooks that provide detailed analysis of intervention strategies, development, and conditions that are available to therapists. The *Handbook* will not replace those resources but rather complement them.

In the first edition of the *Handbook,* we indicated that one of its purposes was to provide critical information to therapists who are expected to initiate interventions with perhaps limited time to research areas in which they do not have a great amount of knowledge. We wanted to help therapists meet the demand of the changing health-care environment and the increasing demand to have a wide breadth of knowledge available. The past 5 years have not diminished that need. In fact, the need has possibly increased as more therapists are moving from some other specialty areas into pediatrics. We hope to assist therapists in finding information quickly so they can enhance their therapeutic expertise.

Although the spirit of the first edition remains, we have made some notable changes that we believe will increase access to the information and readability. We have retained the outline format providing short bursts of information. However, to enhance readability we have reorganized much of the information. The *Handbook* continues to contain six major chapters providing information on key aspects of pediatric physical therapy. As appropriate, we have incorporated language consistent with the *Guide to Physical Therapy Practice.* Because pediatric physical therapy is provided in systems other than those that adhere to the traditional medical or therapy model, we have also included language that is unique to those systems, most notably early intervention and school age services. It is hoped that additional tables, boxes, charts, and figures will increase access to the information. It has always been our goal to limit the need to read through text to capture the essence of the materials.

Based on feedback from readers and colleagues, we have made a few significant changes to the text. The first major change was to separate intervention strategies and pediatric conditions. Because of the complexity of the conditions seen by pediatric physical therapists, there are few protocols available. Rather than repeating general statements related to treatment, we added a chapter on intervention (Chapter 4). This chapter describes the various treatment approaches used in pediatric physical therapy, the philosophy of services provided to children and their families, and where appropriate, specific treatment protocols. We also describe common treatments (such as surgery and medication) provided by colleagues. We have added many more photographs and line drawings to Chapter 5 (Assistive Technology) and have incorporated the development of gait into Chapter 1 (Growth and Development). A bibliography lists comprehensive works that pediatric physical therapists may consider essential sources of current information. Also, an updated resource list is provided containing current Web pages. Our goal remains to facilitate for the reader access to clinically relevant information in a practical format. We hope that this edition is a useful resource.

No book is ever written by the authors alone. Without the support, encouragement, and unsung help of countless people, books would never be finished. First and foremost we acknowledge Britta Battaile, author of Chapter 5, for consolidating the information on assistive technology that has grown incredibly during the past 5 years. Stefan Taske and Jennifer Edelshick are also thanked for completing the tedious job of checking and double-checking addresses, phone numbers, and Web sites on the seemingly limitless resources available to professionals and families. Vernice Thompson is gratefully acknowledged for coming to our rescue and typing, formatting, and reformatting. Very special thanks are also due to Ulita Lushnycky, who steadfastly stayed with this project and who patiently guided it to completion. Without her investment in this project, an uncompleted manuscript would still be stuffed in canvas bags.

Toby Long
Kathy Toscano

Contributors

Second Edition

Britta Battaile, MS, PT, PCS
One Step Ahead
Physical Therapy Services
Bethesda, Maryland

Jennifer Edelshick, DPT
Physical Therapist
Therapy Associates of Martinsville, Inc.
Martinsville, Virginia

Cheryl Levy
Photographer
Bethesda, Maryland

Stefan Taske
Project Researcher
Georgetown University
Child Development Center
Washington, District of Columbia

First Edition

Britta Battaile, MS, PT, PCS
Physical Therapy Services
Bethesda, Maryland

Holly Cintas, PhD, PT, PCS
Coordinator, Physical Therapy Research
National Institutes of Health
Rockville, Maryland

Kathleen Harp, MHS, PT, PCS
Pediatric Physical Therapy
Rockville, Maryland

Andrea Santman Wiener, MHS, PT, PCS
Building Blocks, Pediatric Rehabilitation Services
Washington, District of Columbia

Contents

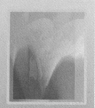

Growth and Development

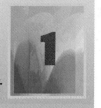

Pediatric therapists are frequently challenged by situations involving children who have problems that represent variations from the usual flow of developmental events. Thorough knowledge of growth and development provides the foundation necessary to identify and analyze differences in development. This chapter describes typical growth and development in children from the neonatal period through childhood. Although an emphasis is placed on the motor system, basic information on language, cognition, and psychosocial development is also presented.

MOTOR DEVELOPMENT

Typical motor development follows a predictable sequence. There are variations in this sequence, and the rate at which each child moves through the sequence varies. Although it may appear that skill development occurs in a cephalocaudal and proximal-to-distal direction and that skills develop from the general to the specific, this does not explain the variability seen in development. The system theories of motor control indicate that there is an interplay among multiple variables that contributes to the rate and variability of development as well as the quality of motor patterns. System theories indicate that children learn functional motor skills through interaction with the environment.

FETAL

Eight weeks' gestation to birth

Motor patterns arise spontaneously and are not reflexive

Anatomic maturation of the arms and legs proceeds cephalocaudally

No gender-related differences have been noted in fetal movements (Table 1-1)

NEONATAL

Birth through 2 weeks of age (Table 1-2)

INFANT

Three weeks through 12 months of age

Development proceeds in a predictable sequence

Sequence can vary in individual children (Table 1-3)

TODDLER

Thirteen months through 2 years of age

Period of increasing independence

Refinement of upright skills

Rapid expansion of language development (Table 1-4)

TABLE 1-1. Motor Development of the Fetus

	10–15 Weeks	17–18 Weeks	20 Weeks
Upper extremity	Isolated extremity movements: hands to face, thumb sucking		Wide arcs of arm movement
Locomotion	Full-body rotation around the umbilicus; climbing on the uterine wall	Vigorous extensor thrusts against uterine wall repositions fetus	Period of greatest motility; creeping/crawling movement
Atypical behaviors	Fetal akinesia	Symmetric, stereotypic movements lacking dissociation	Absent or limited propulsive movements

PRESCHOOL

Three through 5 years of age

Movements become more precise

Skills integrated into play routines and activities

Increasing independence in the performance of activities of daily living (Table 1-5)

 # DEVELOPMENT OF ADAPTIVE SKILLS

Adaptive skills are those activities of daily living or self-help skills that affect the level of independence the child shows during functional tasks

Motor dysfunction can greatly affect a child's ability to perform these activities

There is a large amount of variation in the emergence of these behaviors due to cultural influences and family expectations (Table 1-6)

TABLE 1-2. Movements of the Full-Term Neonate

Position	Movement
Prone	Head elevates to clear face and reposition it; flexor bias of trunk and extremities
Supine	Head rotates fully in either direction but can come to midline with arousal
Sitting	Head may bob while in kyphotic, supported sitting position; head position is typically flexed forward
Upper extremity	Hands fisted much of the time; arms held snug to the body; strong elicited grasp; gross isolated finger movements
Locomotion	May move to side of bassinet while prone
Atypical behaviors	Absence of isolated finger movement; head always positioned to one side; inability to clear face in prone position; exaggerated back extensor arching

TABLE 1-3. Movements Occurring During Infancy

	1 Month	2–3 Months	4–5 Months	6–7 Months	8–9 Months	10–11 Months	12 Months
Prone	Elevates head slightly; rotates head to either side	Elbows in line with shoulders for forearm support; lateral weight-shifting; rolls to supine	Weight-shifting to free arm and reach with one hand	Elevates trunk with elbow extension; may rock on hands and knees; transitions to sitting; pushes backward	Transitions in and out of sitting to quadruped or prone; pulls to stand with support	Pulls to stand by rolling up over feet; pulls to stand through half kneeling	Stands up through quadruped
Supine	Reciprocal kicking alternates with symmetric kicking	Kicking movements	Alternates feet to mouth and bridging; attempts roll to side with leg or arm leading	Brings feet to chin or mouth; rolls to prone; attempts to raise self to sit	Raises self to sit	Transitions to sitting and quadruped	Moves rapidly into sitting or quadruped to standing
Sitting	Forward flexion of trunk; head in line with trunk for short intervals	Midline head alignment; minimal head lag during pull-to-sit maneuver; propped sitting may be emerging	Static ring sitting emerging; attempts lateral weight-shift to support body with one arm and grasp a toy with the other	Static sitting while manipulating a toy; weight-shifting with lateral and anterior arm support	Manipulates toy in sitting position; anterior, lateral protective reactions present	Rotates or pivots while sitting to reach; transitions to prone or supine easily	Wide variety of sitting positions includes side-sitting
Upper extremity	Reaching efforts depend on body position and are linked with visual gaze on an object; opens and closes hands	Reaches and grasps with eye-hand coordination; finger play in mouth	Arms extend fully up in supine to reach in midline; palmar grasp on cube; holds toy with two hands	Brings objects to midline; holds bottle with two hands; rakes for small objects;	Controlled release; transfers objects; radial digital grasp	Pincer grasp	Rolls a ball; scoops with a spoon; finger feeds

(continued)

TABLE 1-3. Movements Occurring During Infancy (continued)

	1 Month	2–3 Months	4–5 Months	6–7 Months	8–9 Months	10–11 Months	12 Months
Locomotion		May achieve a 25–30° arc through pivot-prone rotation; rolls from side to back	Pivot-prone rotation; may attempt rocking in quadruped and pushing backward	Moves forward with arms with or without abdomen elevated	Crawls/creeps; pulls to stand with support	Sidesteps or cruises with external support; walks with one hand held	Independent walking with high guard arms and wide support base; lowers self with control from standing May begin to move in and out of a full squat position
Atypical behaviors	Difficulty flexing legs under body; limited arcs of extremity movement; absence of reciprocal leg movements; no evidence of grasp and release; opistothonis	Inability to right head at end of pull-to-sit maneuver; arching of back	Lateral weight-shifting difficult in prone; unable to extend arms fully and toward midline in supine; kyphotic sitting position; unable to sit erect even with support	Inability to achieve midline head position in supine or sitting; no evidence of movement in prone; inability to tilt pelvis to bring thighs to hands	Commando crawl or bunny-hop; W-sit as the only sitting position	Inability to transition among sitting positions; pulls to standing using arms only; inability to stand on flat feet	Trunk and extremity stiffness, laxity, or instability; poor coordination may prevent hands-knees locomotion and emergence of standing

TABLE 1-4. Motor Development From 13 to 24 Months of Age

	13–15 Months	15–18 Months	18–24 Months
Gross motor	Sustained standing without external support; stoops to pick up object and regains standing; stands from floor without support	Carries or pulls an object while walking; creeps down steps; steps on ball positioned for kicking; tries climbing steps using the railing	Stands on one foot momentarily; steps over low barrier
Perceptual motor	Holds two cubes in same hand; builds 2- to 3-cube tower; hurls objects to floor from table or high chair; flings ball with elbow extension	Turns book pages several at a time; scribbles; builds tower with 3 to 4 cubes; takes pegs from board and attempts to replace	Builds 5- to 6-cube tower; places pellet in bottle; separates pop beads; imitates motor activities
Locomotion	Independent walking; climbs into adult chairs; walks backward a few steps; stoops and recovers easily; carries object while walking, creeps up steps or walks up with external support	Base of support almost equal to width of pelvis; running not well coordinated or with arm reciprocation; walks to the side a few steps	Walks up steps with step-to pattern and external one-hand support; running speed and fluidity increasing; tries to jump off bottom step
Atypical behaviors	Moves around environment using bottom scooting, bunny-hop, or rolling	Lacks independent, upright walking	Base of support wider or narrower than pelvis; falls often while walking or running

■ BIOMECHANICAL INFLUENCES ON DEVELOPMENT

Mechanical forces, mediated by genetic and chemical factors, influence the child's growth from the earliest weeks of development

- Muscle cells grow according to the direction of pull placed on them
- Size and fiber type depend on heredity, age, demand placed on them, gender, and presence of an intact electroneuromuscular apparatus to drive them
- Muscles appear much more compliant than bone to tensile stresses, responding to stretch by lengthening
- Tension forces of muscles on bones are essential to bone development and joint alignment

Rate, shape, and volume of growth of one tissue can determine the magnitude and direction of forces placed on neighboring tissues

Plasticity of tissues can lead to constraint or facilitation of growth in bones and in adjacent tissues

TABLE 1-5. Motor Development From 2 to 5 Years of Age

	2 Years	30 Months	3 Years	42 Months	4 Years	54 Months	5 Years
Gross motor	Kicks small ball forward; throws ball overhand; jumps off low step	Jumps off step with 1 foot leading; jumps off floor with 2 feet; can imitate walking on tiptoes; mounts tricycle	Jumps off step and lands with 2 feet; easily propels riding vehicle with feet on floor, may pedal; jumps over 1- to 2-inch object; positions arms in anticipation to catch a ball	Mounts, pedals, and dismounts several types of 3-wheel riding vehicles; stands on 1 foot for >3 seconds; hops on 1 foot; kicks ball; may jump forward several times in succession	Rotation of body follows forward projection of ball; several hops in succession on 1 foot; stands and walks on tiptoes; rides two-wheeled bike with training wheels	Catches ball by preparing arm as ball approaches, elbows may be at the sides; throws ball to another person 8 to 10 feet away; jumps 2 to 3 inches off the floor	Jumps forward and sideways with 2-foot landing emerging; jumps over object 6 to 8 inches from the floor; throws ball to hit target at 10 feet; roller skates; rides a bike
Perceptual motor	Builds 6- to 7-cube tower; turns book pages singly; turns doorknobs	Imitates straight, horizontal, and circular strokes with marker; tripod grip emerging	Imitates cross-stroke with marker; attempts scissor cut; imitates block bridge building; hand preference emerging	Strings and unstrings beads based on size; builds bridges using blocks; removes bottle cap to check contents	Dynamic tripod pencil grip; makes cross-stroke; attempts to trace line; hand preference is established	Folds sheet of paper in half; cuts large square from paper sheet; beginning to form letters	Dynamic tripod grip; draws simple shapes, letters, or numbers; places small pegs in pegboard and removes them easily; winds string on spool (continued)

TABLE 1-5. Motor Development From 2 to 5 Years of Age (continued)

	2 Years	30 Months	3 Years	42 Months	4 Years	54 Months	5 Years
Locomotion	Ascends and descends stairs alone with step-to pattern; attempts foot-over-foot with adult support	Running well-coordinated with arm reciprocation; walks on line backward	Walks up steps reciprocally; running with speed and fluidity; jumps off bottom step	Runs up to a ball to kick it; may jump with 2 feet in succession	Running fluid with arm reciprocation	Walks on curb or beam without falling	Broad jumps; drop kicks; jumps rope
Atypical behaviors	Not walking or falls often while walking; in-toeing or excessive external rotation; avoids arts and crafts projects; base of support much wider than pelvis or narrowed			Response times insufficient to succeed at catching a ball or soft object; unable to maintain single leg stability to kick, hop, or stand on one leg	Does not attempt skills requiring moderate to maximal balance challenges such as climbing and jumping off heights; catching and kicking balls is difficult; ambiguous hand preference	Difficulty with skills requiring asymmetric body positioning or disassociated extremity movements, such as throwing with one arm, jumping on one leg	Difficulty mounting or pedaling any ride-on toy; often cannot imitate a motor act after seeing another child complete it; base of support wider than pelvis; cannot catch ball; fist grip rather than tripod grip of marker or pencil

TABLE 1-6. Adaptive Skills in Children Ages 18 Months to 5 Years

	18–24 Months	24–30 Months	3 Years	4 Years	5 Years
Feeding	Finger feeds; drinks from cup; scoops with spoon	Uses spoon or fork; pours from one cup to another	Uses utensils consistently	May help set and clear the table	
Dressing	Takes off shoes, socks; holds arm out for donning a shirt	Puts on shoes; pulls pants up and down; finds armholes in coat	Pulls on and removes pullover type clothing	Attempts to button and Unbutton	Unlaces shoes; buckles; buttons and unbuttons
Bladder/ bowel control	May indicate if soiled; may be dry for several hours during the day	May sit on toilet; wakes from nap dry; using toilet regularly	Uses toilet consistently, few accidents		

Movement is essential for complete joint development
- If prenatal movement is diminished or absent, the stress on the joints is diminished; thus, joint dysplasias may develop and lead to contracture or dislocation
- Diminished stress provided by muscle pull over several years has significant impact on leg length and ultimate height of children with lower extremity paralysis

Bone tissue is highly dynamic
- Grows in length and by opposition
- Interior reabsorption occurs simultaneously in response to hereditary, mechanical, nutritive, and hormonal influences
- Wolff's law describes association between bone structure and mechanical demands placed on it
  - Moderately high, consistent mechanical stresses increase bone density
  - Exceedingly high or low mechanical forces on bone result in reabsorption and decreased bone density
- The same quality that underlies transition from mesenchymal membrane (intramembranous ossification) or cartilage (endochondral ossification) to bone allows it to be molded by tension, compression, and torsional forces, especially those exerted by muscles
  - Weight-bearing affects bone growth and alignment
  - Muscle tension on bone is needed to maintain density due to wrapping or positioning
  - Examples of bone molding include skull elongation and foot molding

Forces appear to have a much greater impact on lower than upper extremity development
- The legs are subject to much greater prenatal uterine constraint compared with the arms
- Lower extremities carry the body weight and maintain erect position during growth, placing much more stress on them and increasing the tendency for malalignment over time
- Both hip joints and ankle joints have multiple axes of motion
- Influence of malalignment forces on adjacent joints is greater in a closed kinetic chain

There is a predictable developmental sequence of the relationships between major joint components of the lower extremity (Table 1-7)

TABLE 1-7. Developmental Progression of the Femur

	Age	Mean	Range
Femoral neck–shaft angle	16 weeks GA	140°	130–150°
	32 weeks GA	128°	112–143°
	Birth	135°	118–144°
	1–3 years	145°	131–148°
	4–5 years	135°	123–143°
	9–13 years	135°	121–148°
	15–17 years	130°	121–148°
	Adult	125°	114–140°
Femoral version	16 weeks GA	12° anteversion	15° retroversion–30° anteversion
	32 weeks GA	28°	10–55° anteversion
	Birth	30°	15–55°
	1–3 years	35°	20–50°
	4–5 years	25°	19–38°
	10–12 years	25°	10–35°
	13–20 years	14°	5° retroversion–33° anteversion
	Adult	15°	25° retroversion–35° anteversion
Tibiofemoral angle	Birth	16° varus	34° varus–0° valgus
	6 months	12° varus	
	1 year	10° varus	21° varus–13° valgus
	20 months	0°	
	2 years	2° valgus	
	30 months	8° valgus	20° varus–20° valgus
	3 years	10° valgus	
	4 years	9° valgus	
	5 years	7° valgus	13° varus–19° valgus
	6 years	6° valgus	4° varus–17° valgus
	7–13 years	5° valgus	0° varus–11° valgus
			0° varus–11° valgus
			0° varus–14° valgus

GA, gestational age.

VARIATIONS IN JOINT ALIGNMENT

Trunk

Scoliosis and kyphoscoliosis

- May develop prenatally due to wedge-shaped vertebral bodies or fused vertebrae
- More commonly related to asymmetric muscle pull or lack of support of the trunk
- Conditions that affect motor control can contribute to the development of atypical trunk alignment such as cerebral palsy, spina bifida, spinal muscular atrophy, poliomyelitis, osteogenesis imperfecta, and muscular dystrophies (Table 1-8)

TABLE 1-8. Variations in the Alignment of the Trunk			
	Description	**Intervention**	**Pathology**
Pectus carinatum	Sternum elevated; chest has increased anterior-posterior dimensions	Improves with time and growth; no intervention in mild to moderately severe cases; surgery for cosmetic reasons in extreme instances	Fetal compression during gestation
Pectus excavatum	Sternum depressed relative to adjoining ribs	Identify and remediate cause of respiratory insufficiency; no specific intervention in mild to moderate cases; activation of abdominal musculature to elongate rib cage may have some value	Gestational compression; shortened chorda tendineae of the diaphragm; chronic respiratory insufficiency, especially inspiratory stridor in premature infants
Kyphosis	Anterior curvature; accompanied by forward or hyper-extended head; thoracic or lumbar areas most common	Usually preventable by good attention to postural alignment by caregivers and selection of adaptive devices that promote best alignment	Usually due to atypical muscle tone or paralysis; occasionally due to skeletal disease
Scoliosis	Lateral curvature that may be accompanied by abnormal anterior-posterior alignment and vertebral and rib rotation; may be C-curve or S-curve; may be functional (flexible) or structural (inflexible)	Close attention to alignment, especially in supine and static sitting; exercises for general strengthening, elongation, and respiratory capacity; wide range of bracing, electrical stimulation, and surgical options; bracing or electrical stimulation indicated at 25°, surgery at 40°	Congenital: fetal positioning and confinement Neuromuscular: unbalanced mechanical forces due to paralysis or skeletal maldevelopment Idiopathic: predisposing factors not obvious

Lower Extremity
Hip
Coxa valga: increased angle of inclination of the femoral neck relative to the femoral shaft in the frontal plane

- Approximately 150° at birth

- Decreases with weight-bearing and balanced muscle pull to 125–130° by adulthood
- Abnormal stresses negatively influence acetabular development and may contribute to increased incidence of hip dislocation

Coxa vara: decreased angle of inclination of the femoral neck relative to the femoral shaft in the frontal plane to <125°

- Decreased pressure on acetabulum and increased bending stress on femoral neck lead to predisposition for femoral neck fractures and slipped capital femoral epiphysis

Femoral anteversion: anterior rotation (version or torsion) in the transverse plane of the upper femur relative to the femoral condyles

- Exceeds 25° in the infant and young child
- Decreases to 15° in the adult with growth, balanced muscle pull, and weight-bearing
- Infantile anteversion is frequently maintained in the growing child with spastic cerebral palsy, contributing to in-toeing gait pattern and potential subluxation/dislocation
- In absence of spasticity, often associated with compensatory lateral tibial torsion
- In presence of spasticity, often associated with medial tibial torsion, ankle pronation, and difficulty achieving functional hip external rotation

Femoral retroversion: posterior rotation in the transverse plane of upper femur relative to femoral condyles to <15° anteversion

- Rarely a drawback for the average person, although occasionally accompanied by compensatory medial tibial torsion (Table 1-9)

Knee
Genu valgus, varus: increased lateral (valgus) or medial (varus) knee (tibiofemoral) angulation in the frontal plane

- May be due to hamstring, quadriceps, hip adductor, or hip abductor weakness or spasticity
- Frequent contributors are joint disease or loss of ligamentous integrity, rather than muscle imbalance

Tibial rotation: tibia rotates medially or laterally in relation to femur at the knee joint

- Very common in neonates
- Often due to ligamentous laxity but can result from unbalanced muscle pull, especially medial rotation associated with medial hamstring spasticity and/or ankle pronation, hip anteversion
- Tibial rotation more common than tibial torsion in children with spina bifida

Tibial torsion: rotation medially or laterally within the tibial shaft leading to spiral development of the bone

- Medial torsion typically associated with muscle imbalance of knee-ankle and ankle-foot muscles, especially in children with spastic cerebral palsy (Table 1-10)

Ankle and Foot
Deformities associated with muscle imbalance are extensive (Table 1-11)

■ DEVELOPMENT OF AMBULATION

PRENATAL LOCOMOTION
Repositions the fetus within the uterus

Critical for joint development

Vigorous thrusts off the uterine wall with full hip extension contribute to positioning of the fetus in preparation for birth

TABLE 1-9. Joint Deformities of the Hip

	Description	Intervention	Pathology
Coxa valga	Femur oriented laterally in the coronal plane in relation to the pelvis; dependent on foot orientation during loading; associated with genu varus and excessive hip abduction	May minimize impact on knee development and alignment through use of ankle orthosis; surgery required if hip dislocation is also present	Failure of angle of inclination between femoral shaft and neck to decrease
Coxa vara	Femur oriented medially in the coronal plane in relation to the pelvis; leg shorter on affected side with restricted abduction	Optimize alignment with shoe lift or ankle orthosis, depending on loading pattern and influence on knee	Angle of inclination between femoral shaft and neck <125°; possibly related to muscle pull imbalance
Femoral anteversion	Excessive anterior orientation of femoral neck in relation to long axis of leg; increases hip internal rotation and tendency for in-toeing; often present with medial tibial rotation or torsion in spastic cerebral palsy	Anticipate development of excessive anteversion in spastic cerebral palsy; attempt to balance muscle pull on developing hip and femur through alignment, tone reduction, and muscle activation; surgical intervention occasionally necessary	Rotation >25°
Femoral retroversion	Excessive posterior orientation of femoral neck in relation to long axis of leg; increases hip external rotation and tendency for out-toeing; may be a diagnostic indicator of slipped capital femoral epiphysis in adolescents		Posterior rotation
Femoral torsion	Excessive spiraling may result from insufficient or excessive muscle pull influencing bone growth; often associated with femoral anteversion	Attempt to anticipate and balance muscle forces molding bone; surgical intervention often necessary in severe cases	Spiraling within bone shaft of femur; may be normal in early infant development

(continued)

TABLE 1-9. Joint Deformities of the Hip (continued)

	Description	Intervention	Pathology
Dysplasia/ dislocation	Hip may be subluxed in varying degrees to full dislocation; leg length difference indicative of dislocation; Barlow and Ortolani maneuvers identify subluxation	Congenital: multiple diapers, sleeping position, Pavlik harness, and Frejka pillow; conservative measures before walking; surgery sometimes necessary after 1 year	Congenital: external mechanical forces on joint, especially breech position during late gestation; sloping, shallow acetabulum; laxity of connective tissue in females; fetal akinesia syndrome
	Frequent association with chronic head and trunk asymmetry, exaggerated lower extremity stiffness, and hip abductor spasticity	Muscular: positioning, weight-bearing, and muscle activation; surgical repair of single dislocated hip to avoid scoliosis	Muscular: flaccid paralysis, minimal connective tissue support of the joint
		Movement pattern and tonal imbalance: anticipate outcome in the presence of associated factors; positioning, tone reduction, muscle activation, and early weight-bearing activities	Movement pattern and tonal imbalance: shallow acetabulum and deforming muscular pull on femur

NEONATAL LOCOMOTION

Reciprocal neonatal stepping elicited through pedal pressure in upright

Positive support reaction

LOCOMOTION ABILITIES
DURING THE FIRST YEAR OF LIFE

Birth–3 months: in prone infant will move, sometimes reciprocally to the corner of the crib

3–7 months: pivot prone rotation in which infant elevates and rotates upper body in a circular fashion

5–7 months: sequential rolling or commando crawling

7–9 months: scooting on bottom or hitching, may be asymmetric; hands-and-knees crawling or creeping

8–11 months: cruising; early upright stepping when hands are held

12–15 months: independent walking characterized by short uneven steps, wide base of support, and high guard position of arms; flat foot or forefoot initial contact; increased dorsiflexion during stance; minimal propulsive push-off; 30% of children can increase speed of walk when encouraged to run

TABLE 1-10. Joint Deformities of the Knee

	Description	Intervention	Pathology
Genu valgus	Tibia positioned laterally relative to femur; high association with coxa vara	Ankle orthosis can improve foot and knee alignment; monitor alignment during growth	Medial knee instability; collapsed medial foot; muscle imbalance; degenerative joint disease
Genu varus; tibia vara or Blount disease	Lateral bowing of the tibia; associated with obesity and early walking	May be progressive despite intervention; orthotic efforts first, then surgery	Lateral knee instability; medial growth disturbance of proximal tibial epiphysis
Tibial torsion (exaggerated)	Excessive rotation of tibia relative to femur, spiraling of tibia shaft; almost always medial; frequently associated with equinovarus deformity	Congenital: usually resolves itself with extra diapers to maintain appropriate position	Congenital: rotation forces placed on knee joint and lower leg during gestational compression
		Muscle imbalance: minimize through exercise and bracing such as derotation cables	Muscular: imbalance in muscles attaching at knee joint, especially hamstrings
		Movement pattern: anticipate emergence of internal rotation pattern; muscle activation activities, weight-bearing, and positioning to promote external rotation before achievement of walking	Movement pattern: linked pattern of hip and knee joint internal rotation; associated with femoral anteversion
Genu recurvatum	Posterior tibial glide relative to femur is excessive, especially during standing and walking	Congenital: positioning	Congenital: fetal positioning and confinement, especially breech position
		Musculoskeletal: strength training, positioning, orthosis	Musculoskeletal: joint laxity at the knee or imbalance in muscle strength or activation

TABLE 1-11. Joint Deformities of the Ankle and Foot

	Description	Intervention	Pathology
Metatarsus adductus	Excessive adduction of forefoot with hindfoot neutral or valgus position	Responds to manual stretching and proper positioning; taping or casting	Compression of forefoot when legs flexed across the body during late gestation
Calcaneovalgus	Hyperdorsiflexed foot, often with valgus; associated with hip dislocation	Usually resolves without treatment, but taping may be necessary	Prolonged breech position; uterine position forces foot into extreme dorsiflexion against lower leg
Pes cavus	Abnormally high medial and lateral longitudinal arches accompanied by flexed toes and calcaneovarus	Maintain joint mobility through exercise, especially length of toe flexors; maintain stability through orthotic support	Muscle imbalance often associated with peroneal muscular atrophy, spina bifida, and poliomyelitis
Equinovarus (clubfoot)	Whole foot adduction; often associated with plantar flexion	Almost always requires surgical repair; good outcome if isolated problem, less positive if associated with additional problems	Fetal confinement or fetal akinesia syndrome
Pes equinus (equinus foot)	Chronic calcaneal elevation usually due to shortening of the Achilles tendon; associated with hamstring shortening	Identify contributing factors, particularly role of hamstring and gastroc-soleus spasticity; use back-stepping and sit-to-stand maneuvers to elongate and activate hamstrings and gastroc-soleus; bracing, especially articulated molded ankle-foot orthosis	Imbalance of muscle pull; leg length discrepancy; lpositional in flaccid paralysis; absence of weight-bearing to maintain tendon length

GAIT CHANGES DURING EARLY CHILDHOOD

18 months: heel strike emerges; reciprocal arm swing in half of all children; most children (78%) can increase walking speed

2 years: knee flexion more consistently present during stance phase; some children (7%) can walk a balance beam (10 cm × 3 cm) sideways or with one foot on and one off

30 months: most children toe walk and heel walk; few children (5%) hop forward on one foot

3 years: gait pattern maturing; all components present except for increased cadence and decreased step length relative to adult pattern; running with nonsupport phase emerging

42 months: base of support equivalent to or less than pelvic span

4 years: reciprocal arm swing firmly established; most children walk a balance beam; most children hop forward on one foot

6–7 years: mature gait pattern present with all components, although stride length will continue to increase with increasing height and leg length

TRANSITIONS SEEN IN GAIT PATTERN

Wide base of support decreases to width of pelvic span gradually; can occur up to 3 years after onset of independent walking

Increased gait velocity influenced by increased cadence during transition from supported to independent walking

Increased gait velocity influenced by increased stride length after onset of independent walking

Stride length correlates with age, leg length, and height

Transition from high guard arm position to reciprocal arm swing occurs 4–5 months after onset of independent walking

Transition from flat foot initial contact with excessive hip flexion to heel strike occurs approximately 5–6 months after onset of independent walking (approximately 18 months of age)

Plantar flexion of the ankle with simultaneous flexion of the knee occurs approximately 4 months after independent walking; should be present by age 2

Heel strike facilitated by ankle dorsiflexion in conjunction with knee extension by 2 years of age

COMPONENTS OF AMBULATION

Cadence: number of steps per minute; decreases gradually from toddlerhood to adulthood

- 12 months: 175 steps/min
- 3 years: 153 steps/min
- 7 years: 143 steps/min
- Adult: 114 steps/min

Gait cycle: heel strike on right to heel strike on right

Initial contact: foot strike, heel strike, or heel contact

Pelvic rotation: rotation of pelvis occurring with forward swing and backward stance movement of each leg

Stance phase: 60% of total gait cycle

- Initial/double support: loading period; from initial contact on one foot to toe-off on opposite foot
- Single limb stance: on one foot when other leg is in swing phase

Step length: distance from the heel of one foot to the heel of the other when both feet are on the ground at the same time

Stride length: sum of left and right step length

Swing phase: 40% of gait cycle; begins with toe-off on one foot to heel strike of same foot

- Acceleration phase
- Midswing
- Deceleration

Walking velocity: Average speed in a single direction; dependent on height and leg length more than age

- 12 months: 64 cm/sec
- 3 years: 86 cm/sec
- 7 years: 114 cm/sec
- Adult: 122 cm/sec

ATYPICAL LOCOMOTOR BEHAVIOR

Fetal dyskinesia/akinesia: may be due to neural tube disorders such as anencephaly and spina bifida; congenital myopathies, neuropathies, or encephalopathies; fetal crowding due to uterine malformation or multiple fetuses; insufficient amniotic fluid

Asymmetric or chronic pivot prone rotation: infant rotates to one side only or fails to transition to other forms of locomotion by 9 months; may be due to weakness, inability to weight-shift, or tonal disturbances

Commando crawling: unilateral or bilateral arm-propelled forward movement with trunk in contact with support surface and legs extended; appropriate for child with spina bifida; use of this method for forward movement is a concern if it persists after 9 months of age

Bunny-hopping: quadrupedal, nonreciprocal locomotion using bilateral, extended arms followed by pulling the flexed knees and hips under the body; although all children do this on occasion, it is a concern when the child uses only this method and is unable to transition to other methods or to upright by 18 months of age; typical pattern used by children with spastic diplegia

Bottom scooting, shuffling, hitching: moving forward in the sitting position using arms and heels or legs only; sometimes (although rare) the child will move forward in supine using head and heels; this is a concern if it is the only method of locomotion or if it persists after 12 months of age

Out-toeing (exaggerated external rotation) during stance phase: associated with muscle weakness, connective tissue laxity; may be used to compensate for lack of knee or ankle stability; symptomatic of slipped capital femoral epiphyses (SCFE), especially if unilateral; associated with femoral retroversion or calcaneal malignment; often seen in paralyzing conditions such as spina bifida, polio, lower motor neuron, and intrinsic muscle disorders

In-toeing (exaggerated internal rotation): typical in children younger than 3 years of age; may be due to muscle weakness, tonal imbalance, hip subluxation, increased femoral anteversion, medial tibial torsion, forefront varus, midfoot pronation or supination, calaneal eversion or inversion; often seen in children with spastic diplegia

Genu varus gait: usually corrects spontaneously; if not, can create abnormal forces on tibia or Blount disease

Genu valgus gait: progressive reduction of tibia valgal angle from 3–6.5 years of age; rarely seen after 6.5 years but could be related to severe rheumatoid arthritis

Idiopathic toe walking: may have no relationship to a neurologic or musculoskeletal disorder; may be consistent with sensory processing disorders or in children with significant cognitive impairment

Equinus gait: exaggerated plantar flexion of the foot during swing, forefoot contact during stance; typically due to congenital clubfoot or severely shortened Achilles tendon as a result of chronic muscle imbalance; may stabilize gait in a crouch position; can be an early indication of a neuromuscular problem

Crouch gait: excessive hip and knee flexion, ankle dorsiflexion during stance; may be due to inability to achieve full hip and knee extension due to weakness or hypotonia, hip and knee flexion spasticity

Calcaneal gait: flat-footed gait without push-off that may be due to flaccid paralysis or absence of sensation

Trendelenburg gait: may be due to leg length discrepancy or scoliosis; associated with hip abduction weakness leading to a gluteus medius lurch that may be due to congenital hip dislocation or bilateral intrinsic muscle disease; occasionally due to poor prosthetic fit; may be necessary to advance bilateral long leg braces

■ DEVELOPMENT OF POSTURAL CONTROL

Sensory systems are critical to the development of postural control

Vision appears to be the dominant perceptual means of modulating posture at major transition points during the first year of life: sitting to crawling, crawling to standing, standing to walking

Vestibular system is activated in young infants when vision is occluded and provides feedback on postural orientation

Somatosensory system provides input about limb position

Distal muscles, especially ankle, respond before proximal muscles in children 1–7 years of age in response to perturbation

After 7 years of age, children respond as adults: initially using trunk extensor musculature to maintain posture

■ CULTURAL VARIATION IN THE TYPICAL DEVELOPMENT OF MOTOR ABILITIES

Biologic differences and care-giving practices contribute to differences in motor development that are particularly apparent during the first 2 years of life

Care-giving practices can facilitate either calming effects or stimulation in the infant

Infants of African heritage demonstrate gross motor acceleration

- Motorically very responsive at birth; higher muscle tone and active anterior flexor control
- Care-giving practices emphasize antigravity activities

Infants of Asian and Native American heritage have lower muscle tone at birth

Motor development of white and Hispanic infants is generally between those of infants of African or Asian heritage

Varied locomotor progressions exist in infants and children

- Approximately 12% of children do not crawl or creep before attaining typical ambulation
- Bottom scooting and commando crawling are strategies used by children having no evidence of motor impairment

There are several possible developmental sequences by which children attain ambulation

Varied physical attributes of growing children can affect preferential selection of locomotor behaviors

■ COGNITIVE DEVELOPMENT

Basis for child's problem-solving abilities in multiple domains

Six major processes

- Discrimination: differentiating and grouping things that are alike or different
- Anticipation: expecting a familiar event; related to recognition of patterns and redundancy
- Imitation: copying; enables child to learn new behaviors; facilitates language development
- Object permanence: knowing that an object exists even when not physically present; forms basis for mental representation and use of symbols; serves as foundation for memory
- Attention: concentration on an object or activity; ability to filter out extraneous or competing stimuli
- Problem-solving: mastering a challenge sequence

Initially focuses on self, gradually views self in relationship to others and objects, finally able to represent world with symbols (objects, pictures, words) (Table 1-12)

Infant development tests are unreliable predictors of future intelligence or academic performance

■ SPEECH AND LANGUAGE DEVELOPMENT

Speech: sounds used to transmit information or ideas
- Domains
  - Articulation
  - Resonance
  - Voice
  - Fluency/rhythm

Language: understanding the sounds produced or heard, provide meaning to speech
- Domains develop in a sequence
  - Phonology → Semantics → Grammar → Pragmatics (Table 1-13)

■ PSYCHOSOCIAL AND EMOTIONAL DEVELOPMENT

TEMPERAMENT

Biologically based, consistent over time

Includes child's motor activity level, daily rhythm, moods, adaptability, social interaction, and environmental responsivity

May be a critical influence on child's overt behaviors and responses to interpersonal interactions and intervention strategies

ATTACHMENT

Parent-child attachment is the primary basis for interpersonal relationships

Child's attachment status influences how child relates to environment

Most information available on maternal-infant attachment
- Securely attached infants use the mother's position as a base from which to explore enthusiastically and learn
- Anxious-avoidant infants explore the environment with minimal or no contact with the mother
- Anxious-resistant infants are passive and show great reluctance to separate from the mother; high correlation with low birth weight, low Apgar scores, motor immaturity, and self-regulatory problems

TABLE 1-12. Cognitive Development

0–6 Months	6–12 Months	12 Months	2 Years	3 Years	4 Years	5 Years
Responds to the sound of a bell, rattle	Reaches, inspects, and attends to objects and others	Imitates putting objects in a box	Joins in nursery rhymes and songs	Knows sex of self	Follows 3-stage command in proper order	Appreciates past, present, and future
Prefers patterns	Imitation begins	Understands and follows simple commands	Matches familiar objects	Can point to tongue, neck, arm, knee, thumb	Can name materials objects are made of	Can define six words
Eyes follow a moving person	Responds to own name	Labels one object	Responds correctly to 2 or 3 commands	Tells action in pictures	Gives age	Gives home address, names and ages of siblings
Visually prefers people to objects; recognizes mother	Plays pat-a-cake	Follows one-step directions	Shows and gives names for hair, hands, feet, nose, eyes, mouth, shoes	Has concept of two, three	Knows day, night	Can judge weights
	Waves bye-bye	Points to three body parts (hair, eyes, nose)				Knows names of the following coins: dime, penny, nickel
Associates behaviors and people	Deliberate choice of toy	Identifies pictures in a book (finds the ball)	Sings phrases of songs	Puts together multiple-piece puzzle	Can tell pictorial likenesses and differences	Knows left from right
Repeats action for own sake	Responds to "no-no"	Points to parts of a doll on request	Associates use with objects	Shows appreciation of past and present	Selects heavier weight	Names body parts: palm, eyebrow, elbow, thumb
Vocalizes at mirror image	Simple problem-solving: pulls bell to ring, squeezes doll to make it squeak	Discriminates 2 items —cup, plate, box	Enjoys simple stories read from a picture book	Comprehends three prepositions: on top of, under, inside	Can make opposite analogies	Knows some letters
	Looks at pictures in a book		Gives use of object			

(continued)

TABLE 1-12. Cognitive Development (continued)

0–6 Months	6–12 Months	12 Months	2 Years	3 Years	4 Years	5 Years
Turns head to look for fallen object	Object permanence present		Recognizes self when shown photographs	Tells a simple story	Matches and names four primary colors	Can count to 20
Lengthy inspection of objects in environment	Transfers objects one hand to another		Repeats two digits	Repeats nursery rhymes	Defines pencil, spoon, and car in terms of usage	
			Listens to musical instruments	Knows concepts: big/little, fast/slow, up/down	Listens eagerly to stories	
				Follows a 2-stage command	Follows directions: on, under, in front of, behind	

TABLE 1-13. Language Development

0–6 Months	6–12 Months	12–24 Months	2 Years	3 Years	4 Years	5 Years
Primary purpose of speech mechanism is for breathing	Motor responses accompany vocalizations	Receptive language greater than expressive language	Rapid increase in language growth	Acquires adult syntax and grammar	Questions other's activity	More sophisticated use and comprehension of language
Responds to other's voices	Vocalization used for attention-getting, socialization	Beginning of primitive grammatical system	Demands response from others	Is versatile in language use	Girls exceed boys in linguistic ability at 4.5 years	Increased speech in social interaction
Babbling, coos, gurgles, sounds of contentment	Recreation of sounds to recall a pleasurable situation or object	Frequent repetition of words and syllables	Two-word utterances	Can be controlled by language	Imitation of parents' intonation pattern	Vocabulary of 2000 words
Monosyllabic utterances (0–3 months)	Responds to human speech by smiling and vocalizing	Use of nouns, few verbs, and some adult pronouns	Inflections (latter part of second year)—primitive grammar	Laughs, sighs	Voice well modulated and firm	
Vocalizes pleasure, displeasure	Distinguishes angry and pleasant sounds	20- to 100-word vocabulary	250-word vocabulary	Uses normal loudness and tone	More complicated sentence structure	
Reacts to sounds	Beginning of imitation of parental utterances	Naming of objects in books		900-word vocabulary		
				Use of language in imaginative play		

(continued)

TABLE 1-13. Language Development

0–6 Months	6–12 Months	12–24 Months	2 Years	3 Years	4 Years	5 Years
Smiles at mother's voice	Single words emerging			Self-centered explanations	Vocabulary continues to increase	
Disyllabic utterances (3–6 months)	By 12 months comprehends many nouns and verbs					
	First words (dada, mama, bye-bye)					

MOTIVATION

Child is an active seeker of stimulation, motivated to explore and gain environmental mastery

Basis for goal-oriented behavior

Nurtured by responses to infant's earliest attempts to interact with the environment; child learns that outcomes are contingent on his or her initiation

Child's self-perception of limited influence on environmental outcomes may be basis for lack of motivation

PERSPECTIVES ON PSYCHOSOCIAL AND EMOTIONAL DEVELOPMENT

Cognitive development: Jean Piaget

- Systematically recorded observations of children's cognitive behavior which have been confirmed in societies all over the world
- Organized cognitive development into a sequence of ordinal stages from the infant's need to directly interact with the environment (sensorimotor stage) to the individual's ability to manipulate abstract concepts in the absence of direct experience (formal operational stage)
- Basic premise is that children's mental representations of the world become more sophisticated in proportion to their widening radius of experience (Table 1-14)

Child development in the context of family: Anna Freud

- Emphasis on influence of family dynamics on child development and critical need to view child in the context of the family

Child development in the context of society: Erik Erikson

- Expanded Anna Freud's emphasis on family interaction to human development in the context of cultural influences on the individual
- Developed an ordinal sequence for psychosocial growth based on progression through specific critical junctions, outcomes of which influenced subsequent behavioral responses
- Applied concept of epigenetic development: individual's personality forms as ego progresses through developmental stages

▉ PHYSICAL GROWTH

Growth is dependent on the interaction of nutritive, genetic, hormonal, mechanical, and environmental factors

Charts reflecting a child's size relative to norms for growth parameters such as height, weight, head size, and progress of ossification (bone age) are available

Growth charts are also available for infants born preterm and children with Down syndrome

FETAL GROWTH

Insufficient space due to multiple fetuses or uterine abnormality may create joint deformations, especially clubfoot and hip dislocation

Growth deficiency due to constraint in late gestation usually compensated by catch-up growth following birth

Intrauterine growth retardation (IUGR) may result from maternal malnutrition, illness, placental insufficiency, or exposure to toxic agents such as alcohol, heavy metals, or drugs

TABLE 1-14. Stages of Development: Jean Piaget	
Stage	**Characteristic**
Sensorimotor stage (birth–2 years of age)	
Reflex stage	Primitive life-sustaining behaviors present at birth
Organization of percepts and habits	Infant learning that actions affect the environment (contingency awareness)
Primary circular reactions (birth–8 months)	Influence of one action on another action confined to the infant's body
Secondary circular reactions (8–10 months)	Infant's action on the environment generates a repetitive circuit; begins to modify behavior to test and change environmental responses
Tertiary circular reactions (11 months or older)	Infant links isolated behaviors that were secondary circular reactions into a chain; continually varies behaviors to test environment
Sensorimotor or practical intelligence	Infant uses direct experience, principally manipulatory, to gain knowledge of the world; incorporates objects in the environment into action schemes
Preparation for and organization of concrete operations (2–11 years of age)	
Preoperational stage (2–7 years)	Mental representation linked with language; child is focused on perceptual and spatial properties of objects; egocentricity
Concrete operational stage (7–11 years)	Child now understands permanence of matter through transformations: conservation of volume, number, weight, continuous quantity; orders objects, 1:1 correspondence; conserve equivalence with changes in physical arrangement
Formal operations (12 years–adulthood)	Can generalize to novel situations without direct experience; trial-and-error behavior used for generating and testing hypotheses; flexible, abstract thinking unrelated to direct experience; ability to imagine many possibilities inherent in one situation

Infants of mothers with gestational or insulin-dependent diabetes are frequently large for gestational age

Neonatal size typically unaffected by hypothyroidism or growth hormone insufficiency, but thyroid hormone is essential for fetal skeletal maturation

BIRTH WEIGHT

Average birth weight in the U.S. is 7 lb; the range is between 5.5 lb (2500 g) and 9 lb (~4100 g)

Appropriate/average for gestational age (AGA): birth weight between 10th and 90th percentiles for infant's gestational age

Large for gestational age (LGA): birth weight >90th percentile for gestational age

Small for gestational age (SGA): birth weight <10th percentile for gestational age

Low birth weight (LBW): <2500 g

- Full-term infant weighing <5.5 lb is considered SGA and LBW
- Preterm infant weighing <5.5 lb is considered LBW but not necessarily SGA

Very low birth weight (VLBW): <1500 g

Extremely low birth weight (ELBW): <1000 g

Micropremie: <750/800 g

HEIGHT

Nutrition is a critical factor

- Growth deficiency resulting from malnutrition can be overcome to some extent by catch-up growth
  - Growth deficiency due to malnutrition after age 4 can be fully compensated for by catch-up growth
  - Malnutrition before age 4 reduces ultimate stature and is usually not reversible

Very premature infants can achieve average or above-average height

Multiple factors and conditions can interfere with the individual's ability to reach average adult stature

Pediatric Conditions

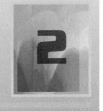

The spectrum of pediatric disorders encountered by physical therapists and other professionals is broad. The diagnosis of a child's condition may encompass several body systems. Most conditions are diagnosed early in a child's life and disrupt development. Other conditions, such as learning disabilities, are not apparent until mid-childhood. This chapter focuses on the incidence, etiology, and essential features of common conditions seen by pediatric physical therapists. Intervention and treatment are discussed in Chapter 4. For the purposes of this chapter, disorders are categorized according to etiology, if it is known. For example, if a disability or condition is known to be due to a specific chromosome abnormality, it will be found under genetics. If a condition has multiple known causes, as does cerebral palsy, it will be categorized under one of the four major sets used in the *Guide to Physical Therapy Practice* (1997); these sets are neurological, musculoskeletal, cardiopulmonary, and integumentary. The category, developmental disabilities, has been added and includes conditions such as mental retardation, processing disorders such as autism, and learning disabilities.

DISRUPTIONS IN TYPICAL DEVELOPMENT

This section contains information about conditions that affect development. Genetic conditions, prematurity, and infections disrupt the normal process of development prenatally, neonatally, or during the first few years of life. Although there is a likelihood that a child may experience a delay, a disorder, an impairment, functional limitation, or disability, in many incidences there are no long-term developmental effects.

GENETIC DISORDERS

Birth defects are the leading cause of infant morbidity and mortality
Account for 30–50% of all pediatric hospital admissions

SINGLE GENE DISORDERS

Mendelian disorders
Occurring in approximately 1% of the population
Caused by error in a single unit of genetic information

Autosomal Dominant

One abnormal gene gives rise to the condition
Generally affect body structures (skin, bone, teeth)

Achondroplasia

Most frequent cause of short stature
Disturbance of endochondral ossification at epiphyseal plate

TABLE 2-1. Types of Osteogenesis Imperfecta

Type I	Type II	Type III	Type IV
Autosomal dominant	Autosomal dominant	Autosomal recessive	Autosomal dominant
Most common	Newborns severely affected; often lethal	Very small in stature	Bones fracture easily before puberty
Bones fracture easily, mostly before puberty	Small stature with small chest and underdeveloped lungs	Fractures at birth are common	Normal sclera
Near normal stature or slightly shorter		Severe early hearing loss	Spinal curvatures
Blue sclera		Loose joints and poor muscle development in arms and legs	Loose joints
Dental problems			
Hearing loss beginning in early 20s or 30s		Barrel-shaped rib cage	
Tendency toward spinal curvatures			

Characteristics may include bilateral shortness of humerus and femur, and macrocephaly associated with hydrocephalus at birth

Forty-six percent of children have spinal complications: kyphosis, stenosis of the spinal canal, or disc lesions

Ectodactyly
Cleft hand or cleft foot in which two or more digits are fused, creating a central opening

Polydactyly
Extra digits present on a hand or foot

Osteogenesis Imperfecta
Error in collagen·development associated with multiple fractures
• Long leg bones are the most frequent fracture sites
• Fractures occur most often between 2 and 3 years of age and between 10 and 15 years of age
• Incidence of fractures decreases after adolescence, although this can be negatively affected by pregnancy, lactation, or periods of inactivity (Table 2-1)

Neurofibromatosis
Slowly progressive disease characterized by an increasing number of tumors with increasing patient age

Usually diagnosed in toddlerhood or early childhood

Approximately 3% of patients have mental retardation; 30% of patients have learning disabilities

Type I (von Recklinghausen's Disease)

Multiple café au lait spots	Scoliosis
Tumors under the skin	Attention deficit hyperactivity disorder (ADHD)
Lisch nodules	Pseudoarthrosis
Glaucoma	Increased risk for malignant and benign tumors

Type II
Bilateral acoustic neuromas
Meningioma
Schwannoma
Neuropathy
Deafness, cataracts

Autosomal Recessive
Both parents are carriers of the gene mutation
Metabolic changes in the blood and other tissues
Occur more frequently in certain ethnic or racial populations

Cystic Fibrosis
Progressive disorder of the exocrine glands
Pancreatic insufficiency
Hyperplasia of mucus-producing cells in the lungs
Excessive electrolyte secretion by the sweat glands
Digital clubbing
Child produces thick, excessive pulmonary secretions that can lead to airway obstruction
    and chronic lung infection
Limited rib excursion, use of accessory muscles of respiration, barrel-chest deformity
Complications include pneumothorax, hemoptysis, atelectasis, bronchiectasis, cor pul-
    monale, and hypertension
Nutritional status is usually compromised

Sickle Cell Disease
Blood disorder related to a defect in hemoglobin which causes anemia
Mostly seen in individuals of African descent
Decreased life span
Affects all major systems
Children may have weakness, pain, and growth retardation

Tay-Sachs Disease
Occurs most often in children of Ashkenazi Jewish descent
Progressive neurologic disorder
Deafness, blindness, and seizures
Development is typical for first several months of life; subsequent rapid progression results
    in death

Spinal Muscular Atrophy (SMA)
Anterior horn cell degeneration and flaccid paralysis
Muscle biopsy and electromyogram (EMG) results confirm diagnosis
Intelligence, social development, sensation, and sphincter function unaffected

SMA I (Werdnig-Hoffmann Disease)
Decreased fetal movements in third trimester, poor head control, hypotonia postnatally
Proximal, symmetric weakness is often identified first, followed by respiratory and feed-
    ing difficulties
Survival beyond 3 years of age is rare

SMA II (Chronic Werdnig-Hoffman Disease)

Has similar patterns of weakness as seen in SMA I but slower progression and more optimistic prognosis

May be evident after 3–6 months of age as motor milestone delay becomes apparent

SMA III (Kugelberg-Welander Disease)

Mild, progressive weakness in proximal muscles

May be evident between 2 and 17 years of age

Differential diagnosis is necessary to rule out muscular dystrophy

X-Linked Disorders

Transmitted on the X chromosome

Males primarily affected; females minimally affected or may be unaffected carriers

Males born to a carrier mother have a 50% chance of inheriting an X-linked disorder; daughters have a 50% chance of becoming carriers

Affected daughter has inherited a mutant gene from both parents; thus, her normal X chromosome has been inactivated

Rett Syndrome

Hypothesized to be X-linked dominant because it is present in females only; lethal to a male fetus

Gradual loss of cognitive, communication, and motor skills; deceleration of head growth; onset of hypotonia; and ataxia after 6 months of age

Often diagnosed initially as autism due to trunk rocking, absence of eye contact, and language disorder

Unique characteristics are stereotyped, repetitive hand-wringing, finger tapping, or mouthing

Fragile X Syndrome

Second most common known cause of mental retardation in males

Older paternal age associated with carrier status in females

Characteristics may include increased head circumference, prominent forehead, generalized hypotonia, torticollis, and scoliosis

Lesch-Nyhan Syndrome

X-linked recessive disorder with excessive production of uric acid and deleterious effect on the brain and liver

Onset of spasticity at 6–8 months of age, subsequent choreoathetosis, growth deficiency, and mental retardation

Metabolic markers for this disorder are detectable by amniocentesis

Distinguished by tendency of children to self-mutilate; may begin with lip-biting at 1–2 years of age and progress to other body parts such as the fingers

Hemophilia

Impaired blood clotting capability leading to bleeding into joints

Hinged joints most typically affected: knee, elbow, ankle

Pain, decreased joint range of motion (ROM), decreased muscle strength

Hemophilia A

Factor VIII deficiency

Hemophilia B
Factor IX deficiency

X-Linked Muscular Dystrophies
Recessive and dominant (Table 2-2)

CHROMOSOME DISORDERS
Occur in approximately 0.7% of all newborns

Account for about 50% of all spontaneous first trimester abortions

Account for about 10–15% of individuals with severe mental retardation and congenital malformations

Most chromosome disorders characterized by mental retardation, unique physical features, congenital anomalies

Disorders on the sex chromosomes characterized by learning disabilities and short or tall stature

Low risk of recurrence in other family members

Chromosome Number Abnormalities
Categorized by number of chromosomes in each pair

- Monosomy: one of a chromosome pair at a specific site
- Trisomy: three of a particular chromosome at a specific site
- Tetrasomy: four of a particular chromosome at a specific site
- Pentasomy: five of a particular chromosome at a specific site

Turner's Syndrome (45 XO)
Incidence in newborn females is between 1 in 3000 to 1 in 10,000

Characteristics may include transient congenital lymphedema, short stature evident at birth, web-like appearance of the lateral neck, underdeveloped gonads, hearing impairment, learning disabilities, and bone trabecular abnormalities

47 XYY Syndrome
Characteristics: tall stature, shoulder girdle weakness, lack of coordination, especially fine motor

Explosive behavioral outbursts and antisocial behaviors

Incidence of XYY syndrome in incarcerated adolescent males is 24 times greater than in the general population of males

Klinefelter's Syndrome (47 XXY)
Present in 1 in 500 males

Most common cause of infertility in adult males

Characteristics: hypogonadism, long limbs, slim stature

Obesity problematic in adults who have not received testosterone replacement therapy before adolescence

Down Syndrome (Trisomy 21)
Most frequent chromosomal disorder associated with moderate to severe cognitive delay

Increased paternal and maternal ages thought to be contributing factors

Trisomy 21 associated with 90% of cases of Down syndrome, remaining cases due to translocation or mosaicism

Can also result from translocation of chromosomal material following breakage

TABLE 2-2. Muscular Dystrophies		
Type	**Characteristics**	**Inheritance**
Neuromuscular diseases		
Duchenne	Onset at 2–6 years; weakness and muscle wasting of proximal musculature; enlarged calves due to muscle being replaced by fat cells; slow progression eventually affecting all voluntary muscles; survival rarely beyond late 20s; Gowers' maneuver often an early sign	X-linked recessive
Becker	Onset in adolescence or adulthood; proximal to distal muscle weakness and muscle wasting; associated with cardiac problems; survival to mid or late adulthood	X-linked recessive
Emery-Dreifuss	Onset in childhood to early teens; weakness and muscle wasting of shoulder, upper arm, and chin muscles; associated with joint deformities; cardiac complications; slow progression	X-linked recessive
Limb-Girdle	Weakness and muscle wasting affecting shoulder and pelvic girdles first; slow progression of generalized weakness; associated with cardiac problems in late stages	X-linked recessive
Facioscapulohumeral (Landouzy-Dejerine)	Onset in childhood to early adulthood; facial muscle weakness with weakness and wasting of shoulders and upper arms; slow progression with periods of rapid deterioration which may span decades	Autosomal dominant
Myotonic dystrophy (Steinert's disease)	Onset in childhood to middle age; weakness and muscle wasting initially affecting face, neck, hands and feet; delayed relaxation of muscles after contraction; slow progression often spanning 50–60 years	Autosomal dominant
Congenital	Onset at birth; general muscle weakness; joint deformities common; slow progression; some children will have severe cognitive deficits	
Peripheral nerve diseases		
Charcot-Marie-Tooth (hereditary motor and sensory neuropathy, peroneal muscular atrophy)	Weakness and atrophy of muscles of hands and lower leg; foot deformities; loss of sensation in feet; slow but variable progression; normal life span	Autosomal dominant Autosomal recessive X-linked recessive X-linked dominant
Dejerine-Sottas disease	Onset in childhood; similar to Charcot-Marie-Tooth but more severe	Autosomal dominant

(continued)

TABLE 2-2. **Muscular Dystrophies** (continued)		
Type	Characteristics	Inheritance
Friedreich's ataxia	Onset in childhood; limb coordination impairments; weakness and muscle wasting; associated with diabetes/heart disease; severity and progression vary	Autosomal recessive
Myopathies		
Myotonia congenita	Onset in infancy to childhood; muscle stiffness; causes discomfort but is not life-threatening	Autosomal dominant Autosomal recessive
Central core disease	Onset in early infancy to childhood; delayed motor development; hip displacement at birth; variable severity and progression	Autosomal dominant
Myotubular myopathy	Onset in infancy; drooping upper eyelids; facial weakness; blackout spells; weakness; slow progression	X-linked recessive Autosomal recessive Autosomal dominant
Nemaline myopathy	Onset in early childhood; delayed motor development; weakness including face and throat muscles; severity and progression vary	Autosomal dominant Autosomal recessive

Mild form associated with mosaicism in which some cells have trisomy 21 and others have normal chromosomal complement

Characteristics: hypotonia, hyperflexibility, excess skin on the back of the neck, flat facial profile, upslanted palpebral fissures, pelvic hypoplasia with shallow acetabular angle, single midpalmer crease

Cardiac abnormalities in 40% of individuals; ventricular septal or artrioventricular canal defects are most common

Hearing and visual defects are common

Orthopedic concerns include atlantoaxial subluxation or dislocation in 12–20%, pes planus, metatarsus varus, scoliosis, patellar and hip subluxation or dislocation

Gross motor delay

Edwards' Syndrome (Trisomy 18)

Second most frequent autosomal trisomy following trisomy 21

Severe cognitive delay

Ninety percent of infants have significant cardiovascular, skeletal, urogenital, and gastrointestinal anomalies and do not survive beyond 1 year of age

Fluctuations between hypotonicity and hypertonicity with increasing age

Polydactyly, finger flexion contractures, and rocker bottom feet

Trisomy 13 (D₁ Trisomy Syndrome)

Limited life span; fewer than 5% of children survive beyond 3 years of age

Severe central nervous system anomalies are common, such as holoprosencephaly associated with anophthalmia or microphthalmia, cleft lip and palate

Polydactyly, finger flexion contractures, and rocker bottom feet

Tetrasomy (48XXYY, 48XXXY) and Pentasomy (49XXXYY, 49XXXXX)

Characterized by decreased stature, hypogenitalism, moderate to severe cognitive delay, and hypotonia

Children with these disorders display many characteristics of Down syndrome

Genetic testing necessary for differential diagnosis

47 XXXY, 47 XXXXY

Severe mental retardation

Multiple congenital anomalies: microcephaly, hypertelorism, strabismus, and cleft palate

Skeletal abnormalities: gene valgum, ples planus, radioulnar stenosis, and malformed cervical vertebrae

Chromosome Structure Abnormalities
Mosaicism

Typically results from a nondisjunction error during mitotic cell division

As zygote cells increase in number to become an embryo, some body cells carry normal chromosomal complement while others have atypical genotype

Occurs in sex chromosomes and autosomes

Children with mosaicism associated with a specific genetic condition have less severe physical and cognitive manifestations than those who are nonmosaic

Translocation

Breakage and transfer of chromosomal material to unrelated, intact chromosome pairs

Occurs in 3–4% of children with Down syndrome; extra 21st chromosome is attached to an intact chromosome other than 21

Basis for other, very rare trisomic syndromes such as trisomy 9, mosaic syndrome

Translocation not always associated with abnormal development; balanced translocation carrier with translocation between chromosomes 14 and 21 may be phenotypically normal with no external manifestation of the translocation

Chromosomal Deletion

Typically induced by chromosome breakage such as translocation, but broken portion is lost rather than reattached

Chromosome breaks that produce translocations and deletions may result from environmental influences such as drugs, radiation, viruses, or chemical teratogens rather than inheritance

Cri Du Chat Syndrome

Results from a terminal deletion of the short arm of chromosome 5

Abnormal laryngeal development results in characteristic weak and high-pitched cry

Cognitive deficit and microcephaly

Hypotonia, hyperterlorism, and scoliosis

Congenital heart abnormalities in 30% of infants

Prader-Willi Syndrome

Source of deletion is paternal

Characteristics include cognitive delay, hypotonia during infancy, short stature, and hyperphagia, which can result in severe obesity

Angelman Syndrome

Source of deletion is maternal

Associated with severe cognitive delay, microcephaly, seizures, ataxia, and frequent laughter

MULTIFACTORIAL DISORDERS

Account for the majority of health defects, chronic conditions, and adult onset disorders

Small variation in genetic information in combination with environmental factors, stress, toxins, allergens, or diet can produce defects

Environmental agents such as radiation, heavy metals, and infectious or chemical teratogens contribute to chromosome abnormalities, especially deletion and translocation, and increase the rate of gene mutations

Multifactorial inheritance occurs when genetic and environmental factors work synergistically to produce anomalies

Environmental factors acting independently are responsible for 7–10% of congenital malformations

Differentiation of inherited disorders from those resulting from an environmental agent is critical for family counseling and prevention of birth defects

MITOCHONDRIAL DISORDERS

Related to disruption in oval-shaped organ cells found in cytoplasm

Affected genes are structurally altered and result in defective energy production

Result in severe adult onset disorders

Mitochondrial Myopathy

Onset in early infancy to adulthood

Characterized by generalized muscle weakness, flaccid neck muscles, inability to work, seizures, deafness, loss of balance and vision, and retardation

Variable progression and severity

Inheritance is through the maternal mitochondrial gene (MT DNA)

PREMATURITY

Birth of an infant before 37 weeks gestation

Infants also have low birthweights, weighing less than 2500 g (see Table 2-3, page 40)

Accounts for approximately 7% of all births in the United States

CAUSES OF PREMATURITY

Many possible causes (Box 2-1)

PHYSICAL CHARACTERISTICS AT BIRTH

Lanugo: fine body hair

Reddish skin color

Lack of skin creases in feet

Lack ear cartilage

Lack breast buds

BOX 2-1. Causes of Prematurity

Chorioamnionitis (amniotic infection)
Drug/alcohol abuse
Fetal distress
Maternal age (adolescent or older mother)
Maternal chronic illnesses
Multiple gestation
Placental bleeding (abruption, previa)
Polyhydramnios (excessive amniotic fluid)
Poor prenatal care
Premature rupture of the membranes
Preeclampsia/toxemia
Uterine abnormalities/incompetent cervix

NEUROLOGIC CHARACTERISTICS AT BIRTH

As gestational age decreases, the following characteristics are more pronounced: hypotonia, hyperextensibility, and poorly developed primitive reflexes

BEHAVIORAL CHARACTERISTICS

Synactive Theory of Neurobehavioral Organization

Hierarchical interaction of four subsystems

1. Autonomic: patterns of respiration, heart rate, thermoregulation, digestion
2. Motor: posture, tone, motor activity of trunk and extremities
3. State: range of states available to infant, transition from one state to another, differentiation of states
4. Attention/interaction: infant's ability to assume and maintain an alert state, respond appropriately to environmental input (Box 2-2)

BOX 2-2. Behavioral Characteristics of Infants Born Prematurely

Younger than 30 weeks postconceptual age
  Remains mostly in a drowsy or sleepy state, little capacity to alert
  Unstable physiologic signs
  Flaccid muscle tone, few elicited responses, and jitteriness
30–34 weeks postconceptual age
  Longer periods of alertness, alternating with drowsiness and fussiness
  Becoming physiologically more stable
  Disorganized movements: kicking, hand-swiping (hand to mouth), scooting to crib corner
  Attends briefly to a caregiver
Older than 34 weeks postconceptual age
  Neither shuts down nor becomes totally disorganized in the face of external stimuli
  Cries or squirms in response to inappropriate stimuli
  Is able to be comforted and cuddles
  Attends to interactions with caregivers

MAJOR COMPLICATIONS OF PREMATURITY

Neuropathologic Conditions

28–32 weeks is the key time for neurologic damage to occur due to vulnerability of the brain and developing glial cells

Intraventricular Hemorrhage (IVH)

Bleeding in the area around lateral ventricles

- Grade I: hemorrhage in germinal matrix only
- Grade II: bleeding within ventricle without distension
- Grade III: bleeding with ventricular dilation
- Grade IV: bleeding extends into brain parenchyma with hydrocephalus

Outcome favorable for children with grades I and II

Children with grades III and IV are at an increased risk for developmental delays and neurologic impairment.

Periventricular Leukomalacia (PVL)

Necrosis of white matter surrounding lateral ventricles

Due to decreased oxygenation and blood flow to the brain

Usually results in spastic diplegia, but with severe and extensive damage can lead to quadriplegia

Seizures

Associated with neurologic dysfunction (IVH, meningitis, sepsis)

Subtle variations in behavior

- Tremors
- Fluttering of eyelids
- Flailing arms/legs

Respiratory Conditions

Respiratory Distress Syndrome (RDS)

Approximately 20% of all premature infants develop RDS during the first or second day of life; rate increases with decreasing gestational age

Caused by immaturity of lungs and lack of surfactant

Survival rate approximately 90%

Treatment

- Surfactant replacement
- Supplemental oxygen

Less than 15% develop severe developmental disability

Bronchopulmonary Dysplasia (BPD)

Chronic lung disease due to long-term need for mechanical ventilation

Walls of lungs thicken, making O_2/CO_2 exchange difficult

Treatment

- Artificial ventilation
- Bronchodilators
- Diuretics

Consequences
- Limited tolerance for physical activity leading to developmental difficulties
- Increased caloric requirement and expenditure resulting in poor growth
- Increased risk for developmental disabilities, poor growth, chronic upper respiratory problems

Apnea

Lack of breathing for 20 seconds or more

Very common due to overall system immaturity

Often seen with bradycardia

May be indicative of systemic medical problem (sepsis, anemia)

Treatment
- Caffeine
- Theophylline to stimulate respiratory centers of the brainstem

Cardiac
Patent Ductus Arteriosus

Occurs in approximately 30% of infants

Lack of closure of the ductus arteriosis (connection between pulmonary artery and aorta)
- Due to decreased O_2 level in blood limiting the muscle contraction needed to close the ductus

Treatment
- Indomethacin
- If heart failure develops, PDA ligation

Bradycardia

Slowing of heart rate to less than 100 beats/min

Associated with apnea

System Immaturity
Hyperbilirubinemia

Accumulation of excess bilirubin in blood

Immature liver unable to excrete bilirubin

Kernicterus

Bilirubin accumulation in basal ganglia which can lead to athetoid cerebral palsy

Necrotizing Enterocolitis (NEC)

Infection of gastrointestinal tract

Occurs in 2–5% of very-low-birthweight (VLBW) infants

Mortality rate is 20%

Factors contributing to ischemic injury to intestinal wall: bacteria, too early introduction of oral formula feeding, bowel immaturity

Treatment
- Antibiotics, intravenous feeding
- Fifty percent of infants will require surgery to remove diseased section of bowel

Gastroesophageal Reflux (GER)

Stomach contents regurgitated into the esophagus

Can last through first 8 months of life (sometimes longer)

Treatment

- Semi-upright positioning
- Antireflux medications

Problems of the Sensory Systems
Retinopathy of Prematurity (ROP)

Abnormal growth of blood vessels that can lead to detached retina

Contributing factor is the high concentration of O_2 used to treat RDS/BPD

Risk increases with decreasing birthweight

Significantly decreased incidence with the advent of cyrotherapy, laser therapy, and improved ventilators

Hearing Impairment

Occurs in 2–5% of VLBW infants

Sensorineural Hearing Loss

Damage to cochlea and vestibular apparatus

Can be due to antibiotics given prophylactically to prevent sepsis

DEVELOPMENT OF THE INFANT BORN PREMATURELY
General Development

There are many differences seen between premature and full-term infants (Table 2-3)

Sensory System Development

Sensory system development is described in Table 2-4

Neuromotor Development

Reflex: by 28 weeks, reflexes are present but are not easily elicited or as robust as seen in a term infant, even at 40 weeks postconceptual age

Muscle tone: hypotonic

- <28 weeks: flaccid, extensor posture
- 32 weeks: active flexor tone begins to develop in a foot-to-head pattern

Motor Activity
Neonatal

Random, disorganized movements

Lack axial tone (Table 2-5)

Through First Year of Life

Transient neurologic signs

- Fluctuating tone
- Irritability or lethargy
- Poorly differentiated reflexes
- Unsophisticated movement components
- Lacks disassociation
- Slowly developing postural control, especially anterior flexor ability
- Predominance of extension

TABLE 2-3. Comparison of Premature and Full-Term Infants*

Premature	Full Term
Physical growth and appearance	
Weight: <2500 g	Weight: 3200 g
Length: 46 cm	Length: 50 cm
Little subcutaneous fat	Much subcutaneous fat, developed over last 2 months of gestation
Narrowed head	Rounded head
Takes up to 2 years to "catch-up"	"Fat pads" in cheeks help strengthen sucking ability
Behavior	
Responds minimally; tires easily	Orients to stimulus in a controlled and modulated manner
Signals difficult to read; poor state control	
Decreased attention	Awake for up to 5 hours
More excitable, restless	
Incoordination of suck-swallow-breathing	
Sensory	
Visual	
Doll's reflex present; prefers human face; follows an arc	Prefers human face; brightens; tracks horizontally
Auditory	
Increase in movement and heart rate in response to sound	Increase in movements followed by habituation
Tactile	
Less behavioral responsiveness in response to touch; hypoactive gag reflex	Behavioral response and increase in heart rate to light touch
Vestibular	
Responds positively to movement	Soothing, is effective to reduce crying
Motor	
Reflexes	
Less robust	Quick, observable, consistent
Muscle tone	
Hypotonic	Within normal limits
Range of motion	
Increased extensibility	Physiologic flexion
Resting posture	
Abduction and external rotation of shoulders, hips	Flexion; abduction; midline orientation
Active movements	
Large amplitude; variable; disorganized	Controlled; less variability; midline movements

*Full-term is defined as birth at 40 weeks postconceptual age.

TABLE 2-4. Sensory System Development

	Age	Behavior
Tactile	8–10 weeks	Responds to tactile stimulation; stimulates self tactilely
Vestibular	28 weeks	Anatomically mature; responds to self-induced movement and externally induced movement
Visual	<30 weeks	Unmodulated eye movements
	32 weeks	Focus briefly on stable object 6–9 inches from face
	33 weeks	Horizontal tracking
	34 weeks	Visual preference; high contrast, complex, curved, human
	35 weeks	Vertical tracking
	38 weeks	Fixates
Auditory	<30 weeks	Avoidance reactions
	36 weeks	Will alert to novel sound

TABLE 2-5. Neonatal Motor Development of the Infant Born Prematurely

	Prone	Supine	Sitting	Hand and Arm	Atypical Behaviors
24 weeks	Very low muscle tone	Extensor bias; low tone; extension, external rotation, and abduction of legs	Unstable physiologic responses, especially cardiorespiratory	Jittery movements, especially distal; elicited responses are primarily avoidant or disorganized	
30 weeks	Longer periods of alertness; minimal crawling behavior	Extensor bias; disorganized kicking	No ability to right in sitting, still some physiologic instability	Hand-swiping; hand-to-mouth; self-comforting movements	Little or no spontaneous movement; cardiorespiratory instability
35 weeks	Head elevates to bob and clear face; quadruped movements	Temporal linkage emerging among hip, knee, ankle during kicking	No evidence of self-support or righting in supported sitting	Hand-to-face and hand-to-mouth movements better controlled	Poor or absent sucking; little spontaneous movement; inability to interact with caregivers

Motor Skill Development

In addition to delayed milestone acquisition, there are qualitative differences in motor performance in children born preterm due to transient neurologic signs, severity of illness and type of neonatal complications, and early neuromotor bias (increased extension, retraction, and elevation of shoulder—scapular region and poorly developed anterior flexor control) (Table 2-6).

Developmental Outcome

Developmental outcomes of children born prematurely are shown in Box 2-3

DISORDERS OF GROWTH

FAILURE TO THRIVE (FTT)

Growth deficiency occurring during infancy and early childhood

Length, weight, and height usually below the 3rd percentile for age

Attributable to psychosocial or biologic factors

Organic and environmental factors may interact

Gastrointestinal or neurologic disorders, or both, are primary organic sources of FTT

Central nervous system (CNS) impairment may result in low responsiveness, poor feeding patterns, and malnutrition

In some children, GER results in decreased nutritional intake

Psychosocial factors should be considered in children younger than 2 years of age who are low weight for length and have no evidence of organic disease

Environmental contributors include inadequate nutrition, inconsistent parenting, and environmental neglect

Evidence of organic disease is present in less than 50% of children typically diagnosed with FTT

Hypothyroidism, hypopituitarism, severe cardiovascular or renal disease, and fetal alcohol syndrome may contribute to growth failure

Growth deficiency associated with cystic fibrosis; elevated sweat electrolytes may also be present in children with nonorganic failure to thrive

Severe FTT is associated with acquired immune deficiency syndrome (AIDS)

DISORDERS ASSOCIATED WITH EXCESSIVE HEIGHT (TABLE 2-7)

These disorders are discussed in Table 2-7

DISORDERS ASSOCIATED WITH SHORT STATURE (TABLE 2-8)

These disorders are discussed in Table 2-8

INFECTIONS

INTRAUTERINE INFECTIONS

May cause fetal malformations

Often go undetected until birth

TABLE 2-6. Comparisons of Postural and Motor Development in the Premature and Full-Term Infant During the First Year of Life

Age	Position	Full-Term	Preterm
4 weeks	Prone	Dominated by flexion	Dominated by extension
	Sitting	Head in midline, arms by side	Very rounded back, forward head
8 weeks	Prone suspension	Head in line with body	Complete flexion
4 months	Sitting with slight support	Back straight; head erect	Needs more support in sitting; scapular retraction; forward head position; fisting
5 months	Prone on elbows	Shoulder-scapula co-contraction; back extension; head upright	Difficulty pushing up and maintaining position; minimal back extension with head in line with trunk
6 months	Prone	Weight on pelvis; lateral weight-shifting	Weight taken on lower rib cage; minimal head righting
	Supine	Sufficient abdominal and leg strength to lift pelvis, activate abdominals, and reach for feet	No lifting of pelvis; when reaching for knees, abdominals do not stabilize pelvis
	Rolling	Supine to prone with rotation	Emergence of lateral righting; may roll with hyperextension of back
	Sitting	Back straight, arms free, beginning to shift weight laterally in preparation for transitions	Propped with back rounded; lack of lateral weight shift
	Standing	Bears weight in standing with wide base; grading of flexion and extension	Minimal weight bearing: often up on toes, stiffening of lower extremities or extremely wide base
	Forward progression	Crawls on all fours; trunk even	If crawling, wide base between knees; lordosis; shoulder elevation
9 months	Supported standing	Base of support narrows; rotates trunk; arms by side	Lordosis; wide base of support; shoulder retraction
	Transitions	Transitions in and out of sitting using lateral weight shifting	Difficulty with transitions due to poor lateral weight shifting
12 months	Upright	Walks (at least with help); base of support narrow	Stands with support; base of support narrow; arms out to side; stiffening of lower extremities; lordosis

> ## BOX 2-3. Developmental Outcome of Infants Born Prematurely
>
> Children born prematurely are at an increased risk for motor difficulties; the risk increases if the child also demonstrates neurologic dysfunction
>
> There is an increased risk for difficulties in visual motor skills even when the child's IQ is within normal limits
>
> Although IQ scores at school age tend to be WNL, group mean scores are consistently lower than standardization samples; children demonstrating subtle neurologic dysfunction are at greater risk for lower scores
>
> Even when IQ scores are WNL, children who were born prematurely use special education services more often than peers who were born full-term; children who were born prematurely also experience more school-related difficulties
>
> Children born prematurely, especially those with documented difficulties in developmental skill performance and/or neurologic dysfunction, are at additional risk for behavior-related problems, especially regarding social competence, activity level, and attention
>
> The risk for cerebral palsy in children born with very low birthweights is 8% (80/1000); the risk in the general population is 0.1% (1/1000)

STORCH
Acronym stands for syphilis, toxoplasmosis, other infections, rubella, cytomegalovirus, and herpes simplex virus

Syphilis
- Maternal syphilis crossing the placenta can lead to treatable syphilis in the infant
- Treatment of the mother before the 16th week of pregnancy can prevent transplacental fetal infection

Toxoplasmosis
- Maternal infection can result from contact with uncooked meat or eggs, unpasteurized milk, or soil or cat feces containing toxoplasmocysts
- Forty percent of children of infected mothers have microcephaly or hydrocephaly, blindness, deafness, mental retardation, or cerebral palsy

Other infections
- Varicella (chicken pox)
  - 25% chance that varicella will pass from mother to fetus, but only 2% risk to fetus for birth defects
  - Defects can include limb, facial, skeletal, and neurologic abnormalities
- Human immunodeficiency virus (HIV)
  - Viral infection suppresses immune system function
  - 90% contract virus from infected mother during gestation, birth, or postnatal period
  - HIV incubation stage may extend several years before development of AIDS; the incubation period is typically shorter in infants and children than in adults
  - Manifests itself in opportunistic infections, failure to thrive, lymphoma, or neurodevelopmental deficits

Rubella
- Can lead to congenital heart defects, vision and hearing loss, microcephaly, mental retardation, and cerebral palsy
- Infections occurring after the first trimester carry a low risk of anomalies

TABLE 2-7. Disorders Associated With Excessive Height

Disorder	Source	Clinical Features	Associated Factors
Beckwith-Wiedemann syndrome	Cause unknown; families in which more than one sibling is affected have been reported	Excessive growth rate in infancy decelerates later; macrosomia; macroglossia	High incidence of prematurity; hemihypertrophy may be present on one side of the body
Fragile X syndrome	X-linked inheritance: fragile site is at Xq27	Growth rate in infancy may resemble cerebral gigantism	Hypotonia, cognitive delay, delayed motor milestones
Homocystinuria syndrome	Autosomal recessive enzyme deficiency resulting in skeletal and visual dysplasias	Failure to thrive with growth deficiency may occur, but normal to tall stature is common; lens subluxation by age 10	Seizures, arachnodactyly, multiple joint malalignment; osteoporosis; mental retardation in most untreated children
Marfan syndrome	Autosomal dominant; connective tissue disorder of undetermined origin	Tall stature associated with little subcutaneous fat, joint laxity with high incidence of scoliosis and kyphosis	Arachnodactyly; normal intelligence; cardiovascular defects such as aortic aneurysm or mitral prolapse may lead to sudden death
Neurofibromatosis	Autosomal dominant with wide variance of expression; multiple system abnormalities	Excessive height may be present in addition to subcutaneous, central nervous system and skeletal tumors	Cognitive deficiency in very few children; seizures; syndactyly; scoliosis; hypoplastic bowing of lower legs
Sotos' syndrome (cerebral gigantism)	Cause unknown; may be autosomal dominant; possible congenital hypothalamic abnormality	Large at birth; rapid growth continues during childhood but final height may be within normal limits	Hands, feet, and skull unusually large; dilated cerebral ventricles; mental retardation
Weaver syndrome	Cause unknown; may be autosomal dominant or X-linked recessive	Accelerated prenatal growth and advanced skeletal maturation during infancy	Progressive spasticity; foot deformities and flexion contractures typical

TABLE 2-8. Disorders Associated With Short Stature

Disorder	Source	Clinical Factors	Associated Factors
Achondroplasia	Autosomal dominant; most common chondrodysplasia; new mutations responsible for 90% of occurrences	Insufficient epiphyseal growth; short extremities, large head with frontal bossing; hydrocephalus and cord compression may occur due to narrow foramen magnum	Early sitting, standing, and walking discouraged to minimize lumbar lordosis and bowing because of weight of large head and proportionately short extremities
Chronic pulmonary disease	Malnutrition major factor; lung disease more significant than malabsorption in cystic fibrosis	Minimal subcutaneous fat; distal digital clubbing with advanced lung disease	Steroidal treatment for asthma may further limit growth
Congenital heart disease	Insufficient tissue nutrition may result from poor cardiovascular dynamics	Growth poorest in children with cyanotic heart disease, but compensatory growth often follows surgical correction	Serum levels of growth hormone same as in nondisabled children
de Lange's syndrome (Cornelia de Lange's syndrome)	Unknown cause	Prenatal onset; short stature; delayed osseous maturation; small limbs; thin downturned upper lip	Motor delay; hypertonia in infancy; multiple joint deformations; cognitive delay; feeding difficulties; seizures
Fetal alcohol syndrome (FAS)	Maternal alcohol ingestion during pregnancy	Prenatal and postnatal growth deficiency; multiple facial abnormalities; microcephaly	Generalized developmental delay; hyperactivity; social immaturity
Growth hormone insufficiency	May be familial: autosomal recessive or dominant, X-linked recessive; may be due to pituitary tumor, especially before craniopharyngioma	High incidence of perinatal problems: excessive vaginal bleeding during gestation, breech delivery, perinatal asphyxia	High-pitched voice; immature facies; excessive breast and abdominal fat; treat with synthetically produced growth hormone before epiphyseal fusion
Hypochondroplasia	Autosomal dominant, but the majority of cases results from new mutations when parents are unaffected	Marked shortening of long bones; normal craniofacial appearance; bowing of legs, milder than achondroplasia	Rare occurrence compared with achondrodysplasia, but incidence of cognitive deficit much higher than achondroplasia

(continued)

TABLE 2-8. Disorders Associated With Short Stature (continued)

Disorder	Source	Clinical Factors	Associated Factors
Celiac disease, Crohn's disease	Nutritional deficiency due to malabsorption; hypopituitarism may coexist	Proportionally small stature that can be compensated if intervention occurs before puberty	Growth may be enhanced by successful steroidal therapy or surgical intervention
Metaphyseal chondroplasia	Autosomal recessive; irregular scalloped metaphyses; gastrointestinal malabsorption is often an early problem that resolves with time	Short stature due to short extremities; fine, sparse hair; joint hypermobility, although elbow flexion contractures are common	Susceptible to chicken pox, which could be fatal due to a cellular immune deficit
Metaphyseal dysostosis	Autosomal dominant; insufficient mineralization of primary calcification areas in the metaphyses	Severe short stature, postnatal onset, limited if any craniofacial involvement; flexion deformities of joints	Waddling gait, deafness may be present
Rickets	Vitamin D deficiency or X-linked vitamin D-resistant rickets (X-linked dominant) or pseudo-vitamin D deficiency rickets (autosomal recessive)	Growth deficiency secondary to hypophosphatemia, hypocalcemia, perhaps insufficient absorption of calcium, phosphorous through intestinal tract	Bowing of legs, coxa vara, hypotonia, fractures; vitamin deficiency rickets and pseudo-vitamin deficiency rickets respond to high doses of vitamin D
Seckel's syndrome	Autosomal recessive inheritance	Prenatal onset of severe growth deficiency, associated with microcephaly, micrognathia, prominent nose	Moderate to severe cognitive deficit, although early motor progress may be near normal; at risk for joint deformations
Silver-Russell syndrome	Unknown cause; may be tentative diagnosis for any infant who is small for gestational age	Prenatal onset of small stature; limb asymmetry common, triangular face, 5th finger incurvation	Motor delay common, although intelligence is usually normal; gradual improvement in growth approaching adulthood
Turner's syndrome (XO syndrome)	45, XO genetic complement or mosaic pattern such as XX/XO; edematous hands or feet may be a marker in the neonate	Short stature, wide neck, broad trunk, lack of breast development; dysplastic ovaries, cardiovascular defects, hearing impairment	Osteoporosis often present related to estrogen deficiency; deficit in spatial ability or visual memory may mask normal intelligence

Cytomegalovirus (CMV)
- Most common cause of congenital infection; occurs in 5–25/1000 births
- Can lead to severe neurologic and sensory impairments, below-average intelligence, behavioral problems, and microcephaly
- Timing of the infection is related to the extent of damage (earlier infections, more damage)

Herpes simplex virus
- Can affect the infant in utero or during birth; infected infants have growth retardation, skin lesions, retinal abnormalities, and microcephaly
- Infants infected during birth can have skin lesions; if left untreated, encephalitis will occur
- Mortality rate is high in infants who are infected during birth and are not treated

INFECTIONS OF CHILDHOOD

Meningitis
Inflammation of the meninges

Bacterial
Most common, caused by bacteria

Meningococcus, *Haemophilus influenzae* type B (HIB)—vaccine

Pneumococcus—vaccine now available

Frequently follows respiratory infection as bacteria live in the mouth and throughout the respiratory tract

Symptoms include fever, stiff neck, vomiting, and seizures in young children

Viral Meningitis and Encephalitis
Less common

Caused by viruses such as mumps, polio, HIV, herpes, and hepatitis

Common in children with leukemia

Gradual or abrupt onset

Symptoms include headache, fever, sore throat, vomiting, back pain, and abdominal pain

Encephalitis is frequently associated with childhood disease; thus, incidence has decreased with widespread vaccinations

Encephalitis is also associated with mosquitoes and ticks; thus, it often occurs in the summer and in tropical climates

■ PRENATAL EXPOSURE TO DRUGS, ALCOHOL, AND OTHER TERATOGENS (TABLE 2-9)

ALCOHOL-RELATED BIRTH DEFECTS (ARBD)

A spectrum of physical and neurodevelopmental effects on the fetus due to maternal ingestion of alcohol during pregnancy

Account for approximately 5% of all congenital anomalies and 10–20% of all cases of mental retardation (leading known cause of mental retardation)

Fetal Alcohol Syndrome (FAS)
Diagnostic criteria are shown in Table 2-10

Incidence: 1–2/1000

Additional physical characteristics: cardiac anomalies, joint, limb anomalies, visual impairments (strabismus, nystagmus, astigmatism, myopia)

Behavioral or emotional disturbances

TABLE 2-9. Possible Effects of Maternal Substance Use

Pregnancy Complications	Neonatal Complications	Childhood Health and Development
Nicotine		
Miscarriage	Low birthweight	Slow growth
Prematurity,	Increased risk of SIDS	Learning disabilities
IUGR	Increased neonatal	Behavioral problems
Preeclampsia	mortality	Respiratory disease during first 5 years
Placental abruption		
Placenta previa		
Alcohol		
Miscarriage	Withdrawal	Fetal alcohol syndrome
Poor weight gain	Low birthweight	
Anemia	Restlessness	
Hepatitis	Poor sucking	
Opiates		
Prematurity	Withdrawal	Developmental delay
Toxemia	High-pitched cry	Learning disabilities
	Irritability	Hyperactivity
	Seizures	Hearing deficit
	Fever	Visual impairment
	Sleep disturbances	
	Diarrhea	
	Tremulousness	
	Poor feeding	
	Vomiting	
	Increased risk of SIDS	

IUGR, intrauterine growth retardation; SIDS, sudden infant death syndrome.

TABLE 2-10. Diagnostic Criteria for Fetal Alcohol Syndrome

Growth Retardation	CNS Abnormalities	Craniofacial Abnormalities
Prenatal growth retardation (less than 10th percentile) or postnatal growth retardation (less than 10th percentile)	Irritability in infancy	Microphthalmia and/or short palpebral fissure
	Hyperactivity and attention impairments in childhood	Thin upper lip, poorly developed philtrum, flat maxillae
	Developmental delays (delay, learning disabilities, mental retardation)	
	Hypotonia and motor problems	
	Microcephaly	
	Seizures	

- Poor judgment
- Oppositional and defiant behavior
- Inappropriate socialization
- Social withdrawal
- Lack reciprocal friendships
- Significantly increased risk to participate in high-risk activity

Fetal Alcohol Effects (FAE) or Alcohol-Related Neurodevelopmental Disorder (ARND)

Incidence: 3–5/1000

Absence of craniofacial malformations

Less cognitive/developmental impairment than in FAS

- Usually have learning disabilities or IQ in borderline range

NICOTINE

Increases risk for miscarriage or low birthweight

Birthweight is dose-related: decreasing birthweight with increasing number of cigarettes per day

May have long-term effects on development such as increased incidence of learning disabilities

ILLICIT DRUGS (COCAINE, OPIATES, MARIJUANA, PCP)

Difficult to determine effects of specific drugs on the fetus because maternal substance abuse often includes multiple drugs, alcohol, and nicotine

Further confounded by prematurity, adverse environmental factors, and genetic effects

Research studies report a range of outcomes from no specific developmental sequelae to CNS impairment; animal studies have shown a wide continuum of effects from prenatal death to subtle behavior variations

Neonatal behaviors may include tremulousness, sleep disorders, poor state control, hyperirritability, and ineffectual sucking

Once infants' conditions have stabilized, developmental scores are typically within normal limits but are significantly lower than matched groups with no history of maternal drug abuse

LEGAL DRUGS/MEDICATIONS

Some drugs or medications taken by mothers can lead to congenital birth defects (Table 2-11)

◼ BIRTH DEFECTS

Birth defects are the result of chance (e.g., fresh mutation, genetic effects, environmental effects, or an interaction of factors)

MALFORMATIONS

Result from primary tissue defects originating within embryo or fetus

Identified genetic disorders account for only about one-third of congenital malformations; remaining are presumed to be multifactorial

Sequence is a cascade of subsequent anomalies that can follow a single, primary malformation

TABLE 2-11. Malformations Associated With Use of Anticonvulsant Medications				
	Dilantin	Phenobarbital	Tegretol	Depakene
Facial	√	√	√	√
Head and neck	√	√	√	√
Limb and digital	√		√	
Growth retardation	√		√	√
Cognitive	√	√?	√	√
Neural tube				√
Cardiac				√
Urogenital				√
Skeletal/limb				√
Skin/muscle				√
Digital (no limb)		√		

Syndrome denotes multiple independent anomalies that develop from one primary cause (e.g., Down syndrome, osteogenesis imperfecta)

DEFORMATIONS

Result from atypical mechanical forces altering normal development

Typically due to extrinsic forces such as intrauterine position or constraint

Occasionally can be a secondary outcome of an intrinsic factor within the fetus, such as a malformation

In general, deformations are far less serious than malformations; most have optimistic prognoses

Oligohydramnios Sequence

Severe form of fetal constraint

Amniotic fluid insufficiency late in gestation due to chronic leakage or faulty fetal urine production

Diminished fetal growth, respiratory suppression, and multiple joint contractures

DISRUPTIONS BY EXTERNAL AGENTS

Cause breakdown of fetal tissues developing normally up to that point

Infectious, vascular, or mechanical

Fetal rubella syndrome and fetal alcohol syndrome are examples of disruptions created by maternal infection or an environmental agent

Mechanical compression of the embryo secondary to premature amnion rupture can result in deformities such as amputation, syndactyly, or scoliosis

CHARGE ASSOCIATION SYNDROME

The CHARGE acronym refers to *c*oloboma or cranial nerves, *h*eart defect, *a*tresia of the choanae, *r*etardation of growth and development, *g*enital and urinary abnormalities, and *e*ar abnormalities and hearing loss

Coloboma: cleft or failure to close the eyeball
- Can result in significant vision loss
- Light sensitivity

Cranial nerves: associated facial palsy, swallowing problems, and sensorineural hearing loss

Heart defect: minor to major defects seen

Atresia of the choanae: passages from the back of the nose to the throat are blocked

Retardation of growth and development
- Small in size due to nutritional problems
- Developmentally delayed due to sensory deficits, frequent hospitalizations
- Some children will have mental retardation

Genital and urinary abnormalities
- Boys have small penis and/or undescended testes
- Girls have small labia; may require hormone therapy to achieve puberty

Ear abnormalities and hearing loss
- Unusual external ears
- Often have short, wide ears with little or no earlobe
- Hearing loss in 80–85% of children

Associated with other birth defects including cleft lip and palate, tracheoesophageal atresia or fistula

Cause is unknown and occurs sporadically

VATER (VACTERL, VATERS) SYNDROME

The acronym VATER stands for *v*ertebrae problems (such as malformed vertebrae, hemivertebrae, extra ribs), imperforated *a*nus, *t*racheal esophageal fistula, *e*sophageal atresia, and malformed *r*adius, *r*enal problems (malformed or absent kidney)

Other letters sometimes used are as follows:
- C: cardiac defects
- L: limb problems—extra fingers or shortened limbs
- S: single umbilical artery

Cause is unknown

▪ CHILD ABUSE AND NEGLECT

Approximately 1% of all children in the United States are abused or neglected

According to the U.S. Department of Health and Human Services, approximately 50% of all reports regarding abuse and neglect of children are for neglect

Children with disabilities are at high risk for abuse

Physical therapists, like all medical professionals, are obligated under law to report suspected cases of abuse or neglect

INDICATORS OF PHYSICAL ABUSE (BOX 2-4)
Shaken Baby Syndrome

Most dangerous in children younger than 6 months

Usually due to frustrated caregiver's inappropriate attempts to calm a crying baby

May result in acceleration injuries, shear forces injuries, coup and contra-coup injuries, and detached retinas

BOX 2-4. Indicators of Physical Abuse

Bruises and welts
  Pattern bruises that resemble the object used to inflict the injury, such as a hand, teeth, belt buckle, rope, or paddle
  Hematomas
  Repeated chronic injuries
  Bruises in multiple stages of healing
  Bruises on an infant, especially on the face

Burns
  Immersion burns indicating being dunked in a hot liquid ("sock" or "glove" burns on the arms or legs or doughnut-shaped burns on the buttocks and genitalia)
  Cigarette burns, especially on soles, palms, back, or buttocks
  Patterned burns that resemble a hot object (burner, iron, grill, heater), especially when on a nonexploratory body surface

Fractures
  Extremities, skull, and rib cage are the most common fracture sites
  Spiral fractures or injuries caused by twisting or pulling
  Metaphyseal or corner fractures of long bones
  Epiphyseal separations
  Posterior rib fractures
  Rib fractures in infants and children
  Multiple or wide complex skull fractures
  Scapular and sternal fractures
  Multiple fractures
  Femoral fractures in children younger than 2 years
  Fractures that do not correlate with the child's gross motor abilities

Lacerations or abrasions
  Rope burns, particularly on wrist, ankles, neck, and torso
  Lacerations or abrasions on palate, mouth, gums, lips, eyes, ears, or external genitalia
  Bite marks

Abdominal injuries
  Rigid abdomen; tenderness in abdomen
  Duodenal or jejunal hematomas
  Rupture of the vena cava
  Peritonitis—inflammation of the lining of the abdominal cavity
  Renal injury
  Injury of internal organs (ruptured liver, spleen, kidney, or bladder injury)

Head injuries
  Absence of hair or hemorrhaging beneath the scalp (due to vigorous hair pulling)
  Central nervous system involvement, which may indicate head injury from violent shaking
  Subdural hematoma (from blunt trauma or shaking)
  Retinal hemorrhage (from shaking)
  Cerebral infarction, secondary to cerebral edema
  Jaw and nasal fractures
  Loosened or missing teeth

Reprinted with permission from Wynn, K. F. (1999). Out of harms way. *PT Magazine, 7,* 42.

SIGNS OF SEXUAL ABUSE

Fear

Shyness

Extroversion

Provocative, inappropriate sexual behavior

INDICATORS OF CHILD NEGLECT

There are many indicators of child neglect (Box 2-5)

 MULTIPLE BIRTHS

There has been a 26% increase in multiple births in the United States since 1970

Twin births now account for l in 43 live births in the United States

The higher frequency of multiple births is due to advances in reproductive technology

Multiple births can lead to premature delivery

BOX 2-5. Indicators of Child Neglect

The following have been noted to be indicators of child neglect. It is important to gather information regarding the individual circumstances of the family to determine if neglect is truly present. In identifying neglect, one must be sensitive to differing cultural expectations and values, differing child-rearing practices, and the issue of poverty versus neglect.

Lack of supervision
  Very young children left unattended
  Children left in the care of other children too young to protect them
  Children inadequately supervised for long periods or when engaged in dangerous activities

Lack of adequate clothing and good hygiene
  Children dressed inadequately for the weather
  Persistent skin disorders resulting from improper hygiene
  Children chronically dirty and unbathed

Lack of medical or dental care
  Children whose needs for medical or dental care, or medication and health aids, are unmet
  Frequently missed medical or physical therapy appointments

Lack of adequate nutrition
  Children lacking sufficient quantity or quality of food
  Children consistently complaining of hunger or rummaging for food
  Children who display severe developmental lags

Lack of adequate shelter
  Structurally unsafe housing or exposed wiring
  Inadequate heating
  Unsanitary housing conditions

Reprinted with permission from Wynn, K. E. (1999). Out of harms way, *PT Magazine, 7,* 42.
Source: National Center for Child Abuse and Neglect, Chicago, Illinois, 1998.

Multiple births occur with greater frequency in older women

Increased risk for developmental problems

- Incidence of cerebral palsy (CP) is at least six times higher in multiple than in singleton births
- Potential for birth defects is related to fetal crowding

Specific birth defects are associated with multiplicity

- Higher than average incidence of VATER syndrome (vertebral anomalies, ventricular septal defect, tracheoesophageal fistula, and radial dysplasia)
- Sacrococcygeal teratoma
- Holoprosencephaly and anencephaly

SPECIFIC CONDITIONS SEEN BY PEDIATRIC PHYSICAL THERAPISTS

This section describes those conditions with known impairments, functional limitations, or disabilities. They have been divided into five categories, four of which are used in the *Guide to Physical Therapy Practice* (1997) (musculoskeletal, neurological, cardiopulmonary, and integumentary). A fifth category—developmental disabilities—covers conditions such as mental retardation, learning disabilities, and processing disorders.

MUSCULOSKELETAL DISORDERS

LEGG-CALVÉ-PERTHES DISEASE (LCPD)

Degeneration of the femoral head from a disturbance in the blood supply

Has a 2- to 4-year progression

Heals eventually

Occurs more often in boys

Majority of cases occur between 4 and 8 years of age

Primarily affects one hip

Mild pain in groin and medial thigh

Decreased ROM, more so in hip abduction and internal rotation

Positive Trendelenburg

Leg length discrepancy

There is an indication that degenerative arthritis of the hip occurs in later adulthood in those who had LCPD in childhood

Associated problems include osteochondritis dissecans, primarily of the distal femur

Stages
The four stages are shown in Table 2-12

SLIPPED CAPITAL FEMORAL EPIPHYSIS (SCFE)

Commonly occurs in preadolescence and early teens, more so in boys

The femoral head slides off the femoral neck due to slipping of femoral epiphysis

Presents with limp and pain in groin, buttock, or thigh following trauma

Positive Trendelenburg if abductors are weak

ROM limitation in internal rotation, abduction

TABLE 2-12. Radiographic Stages in Legg-Calvé-Perthes Disease (LCPD)

Stage	Radiographic Changes	Risk for Deformity
Initial stage	Failure of the femoral head to grow because of lack of blood supply; head appears smaller and medial joint space appears wider than the opposite side	High
Fragmentation stage	Epiphysis appears fragmented; new bone is beginning to form on the old bone; revascularization of the femoral head is occurring	High
Reossification stage	Bone density returns to normal; changes in shape and structure of head and neck	Minimal
Healed stage	The femoral neck and head retain any residual deformity from the repair process	Residual deformity

Adapted with permission from Ratliffe, K. T. (1998). *Clinical Pediatric Physical Therapy: A Guide for the Physical Therapy Team* (p. 83). St. Louis, MO: Mosby.

Types

There are three types:

- Chronic: gradual onset with a progression of symptoms over 3 weeks
- Acute: sudden onset of severe pain, usually precipitated by trauma
- Acute or chronic: gradual onset of symptoms and trauma causing exacerbation

Severity is measured in four grades of slippage

INFECTIOUS DISEASES OF THE HIP

Osteomyelitis: bone infection; most common in children 0–5 years of age; most common site, distal femur and proximal tibia

Bacterial infections such as those due to staphylococcus, *Escherichia coli,* and streptococcus are spread via the blood

Septic joint:

- Can occur with or without osteomyelitis
- Bacterial infection in joint; can cause joint destruction and thus deformity
- The hip is the most common joint

CONGENTAL DYSPLASIA OF THE HIP (CDH)/DEVELOPMENTAL DYSPLASIA OF THE HIP (DDH)

Acetabulum and femoral head not aligned normally

Occurs more often in girls and in the left hip

Associated problems include cervical torticollis, postural scoliosis, facial deformities, metatarsus adductus, and calcaneovalgus

Types

The five types are shown in Table 2-13

TABLE 2-13. Types of Developmental Dysplasia of the Hip	
Type	Definition
Dysplasia	Acetabulum may be shallow or small with poor lateral borders; may occur alone or with any level of femoral deformity or displacement
Subluxatable	Femoral head can be partially displaced to the rim of the acetabulum; slides laterally, but not all the way out of the socket
Dislocatable	Femoral head in socket but can be displaced completely outside the acetabulum with manual pressure
Dislocated	Femoral head lies completely outside hip socket but can be reduced with manual pressure
Teratologic	Femoral head lies completely outside the hip socket and cannot be reduced with manual pressure; deformity of the joint surfaces is significant; usually related to another severe developmental anomaly, such as arthrogryposis or myelomeningocele

Adapted with permission from Ratliffe, K. T. (1998). *Clinical Pediatric Physical Therapy: A Guide for the Physical Therapy Team* (p. 78). St. Louis, MO: Mosby.

TORTICOLLIS

Exaggerated lateral flexion of the head to one side and rotation to the opposite side due to shortening of sternocleidomastoid or muscular imbalance

May be associated with hypotonia, scoliosis

Usually due to in utero or neonatal positioning but also due to visual problems, pseudotumor, hematoma, and birth trauma

ARTHROGRYPOSIS (MULTIPLE CONGENITAL CONTRACTURES)

Joint contractures due to intrauterine akinesia or dyskinesia; may be neurogenic or myogenic in origin

Multiple, nonprogressive, symmetric joint

Contractures in infants, often accompanied by hip dislocation, club feet, and generalized muscle atrophy

Extent and severity can vary

Pattern One

Upper extremity: shoulder internal rotation, elbow flexion, wrist flexion, ulna deviation

Lower extremity: hip abduction, external rotation, knee flexion, club feet

Children often require assistive devices for mobility

Pattern Two

Upper extremity: shoulder internal rotation, elbow flexion, wrist flexion, ulna deviation

Lower extremity: hips in flexion, knee extension, club feet

Associated problems

- Scoliosis, congenital heart disease, facial abnormalities, respiratory problems, abdominal hernias, feeding disorders

JUVENILE RHEUMATOID ARTHRITIS (JRA)

Most common chronic rheumatic disease of childhood

Group of diseases characterized by chronic joint inflammation

Systemic

Multisystem involvement: pericarditis, myocarditis, hepatosplenomegaly

Multiple joint pain

Joint inflammation

Least common form

Polyarticular

Usually unilateral involvement of five or more joints

Most often involve knees, ankles

More prominent in girls

Gait usually affected in polyarticular form

Two groups

Early onset: development of symptoms between 1 and 3 years of age

Early adolescence: development of symptoms around puberty; associated with a poorer prognosis

Pauciarticular

Most frequently occurring type

Involvement in four joints or fewer

Typically hip joint involvement that may progress to pelvis and spine: spondyloarthropathy (Table 2-14)

Limitations dependent on pain and mobility

Two Subgroups

* Females age 4 and older
    * High risk of blindness secondary to chronic inflammation of iris
    * Can include leg length descrepancy, subluxation
    * Can progress to polyarticular form
* Males age 10 and older

LIMB DEFICIENCIES

Causes

Congenital: typically the result of limb maldevelopment occurring at approximately 4–7 weeks' gestation

Amniotic bands: premature amnion rupture and subsequent band constriction around a portion of a limb, interrupting vascular supply

Cancer: osteosarcoma most common bone cancer in children; occurs most often in epiphysis of long bones, primarily femur

Trauma

Genetics: associated with polydactyly and ectrodactyly

Types

Types of limb deficiencies are shown in Table 2-15

TABLE 2-14. Spondyloarthropathies in Children

Spondyloarthropathy	Age at Onset	Description
Ankylosing spondylitis	Adolescence (boys > girls)	May begin with pauciarticular arthritis in childhood or back pain in adolescence; can lead to general arthritis and in severe cases to ankylosis or fusion of the spine; treatment includes drugs similar to those used in juvenile rheumatoid arthritis to decrease inflammation; swimming and gentle exercise to maintain range of motion and strength
Psoriatic arthritis	9–10 years (girls > boys)	Arthritis that involves primarily the distal joints of the hands with psoriasis; usually mild but may lead to general joint destruction; teach joint protection
Reactive arthritis (Reiter's syndrome)	Variable	Urethritis, ocular disturbances, and arthritis; may be a brief illness with complete recovery or may have long-term sequelae
Inflammatory bowel disease	Variable	Arthritis may be the presenting complaint in children with ulcerative colitis or Crohn's disease: abdominal cramping, diarrhea, weight loss, unexplained fever, and pauciarticular arthritis; septic joints, especially the hip, can occur

Adapted with permission from Ratliffe, K. T. (1998). *Clinical Pediatric Physical Therapy: A Guide for the Physical Therapy Team* (p. 119). St. Louis, MO: Mosby.

TABLE 2-15. Limb Deficiencies

Type	Deficiencies
Acheiria	Absence of a hand
Amelia or ectromelia	Complete absence of a limb
Apodia	Absence of a foot
Ectodactyly	Partial or complete absence of a digit; also refers to cleft hand or cleft foot, in which two or more digits are fused, leaving a central opening
Hemimelia or meromelia	Absence of some portion of a limb; refers to mild or moderate limb defects
Intercalary limb deficit	Only the middle part of the limb is affected
Phocomelia	Top portion of the limb is absent, and the terminal part of the limb is attached higher than would normally be expected (e.g., the hand may be attached to the shoulder)
Polydactyly	Extra digits are present on the hand or foot
Proximal focal femoral deficiency	Partial form of phocomelia in which the shaft of the femur is always short, the femoral head may not be present, or there may be no bony connection between the femoral head and shaft
Syndactyly	Digits are fused together

Classification
Transverse Deficiency
A limb has developed normally up to a certain point, and the structures beyond that point are missing; mostly unilateral

Longitudinal Deficiency
Limb missing specific elements in the long axis

Aitken Classification of Proximal Femoral Focal Deficiency (PFFD)
This classification system is shown in Table 2-16

POSTURAL DEFORMITY
Scoliosis
Lateral curvature of the spine with or without vertebral rotation

Multifactorial causes: neuromuscular, orthopedic, congenital, poor posture, idiopathic

Types
Table 2-17 describes types of scoliosis

TABLE 2-16. **Aitken Classification of Proximal Femoral Focal Deficiency (PFFD)**

Class	Description
A	Femoral head present
	Acetabulum normal
	Short femoral segment
	Femoral head is in acetabulum
	Contiguous femur
	Subtrochanteric varus angulation
	May be subtrochanteric pseudoarthosis
B	Femoral head present
	Acetabulum may be dysplastic
	Femur shortened
	Femoral head is in acetabulum
	No bony connection between head and shaft of femur
C	Femoral head absent or represented by bony remnant (ossicle)
	Acetabulum severely dysplastic
	Femur shortened, usually tapered proximally
	Femoral head not in acetabulum
	Femoral shaft and bony ossicle may be connected by bone
D	Femoral head absent
	Acetabulum absent
	Femur shortened and deformed
	No connection between femur and pelvis

Reprinted with permission from Ratliffe, K. T. (1998). *Clinical Pediatric Physical Therapy: A Guide for the Physical Therapy Team* (p. 106). St. Louis, MO: Mosby.

CHAPTER 2

TABLE 2-17. Types of Scoliosis

Type	Definition
Functional	No structural change
	Correctable with forward bending
	May be related to poor posture
Structural	Changes in vertebrae
	Decreased flexibility
	Vertebrael rotation
Neuromuscular	Associated with neuromuscular condition (CP, MD, SB)
Idiopathic	Most common form
	Most common in girls
	Unknown causes
Traumatic	Associated with spinal trauma (fractures, tumors)

CP, cerebral palsy, MD, muscular dystrophy; SB, spina bifida .

Description
Age at Onset
Congenital: 0–3 years
Juvenile: 4–puberty
Adolescent: during or soon after puberty

Severity of Curve (Determined by the Cobb Method)
Mild: 0–20°
Moderate: 21–40°
Severe: >40°

Direction
Apex to left or right

Location
Cervical
Cervicothoracic
Thoracic
Thoracolumbar
Lumbar

Kyphosis
Anteroposterior curve of the cervicothoracic region primarily caused by poor posture
Structural changes include anteriorly wedged vertebrae, narrowing of intervertebrae disk spaces, irregular vertebrae end plates
One-third of children have accompanying scoliosis
Clinical features include forward shoulders, head

Lordosis
Anterior curve of lumbar spine
Severe anterior pelvic tilt

Often has accompanying genu recurvatum

Usually resolves by age 8 when seen in toddlers

■ NEUROLOGICAL

BRACHIAL PLEXUS INJURY

Compression or traction injury to the brachial plexus, typically unilateral

May occur secondary to trauma to the shoulder from prenatal or postnatal events or anomalies such as cervical rib or abnormal thoracic vertebrae

Most commonly associated with a difficult birth process

Symptoms can range from swelling of the neural sheath to total avulsion of the nerve roots from the spinal cord, resulting in the interruption of sensory and/or motor impulse transmission

Electromyography is useful in determining extent of nerve damage; prognosis is related to severity of injury rather than extent of involvement and is favorable in most instances

Fractures of the clavicle or humerus, shoulder dislocation, and facial or phrenic nerve damage may coexist

Sensory impairment is typically present; however, it may not correspond to motor involvement and is difficult to assess in infants

- Response to pin prick useful to determine baseline loss and recovery of function
- Because denervated skin does not wrinkle in water, the presence of wrinkles after the "wrinkle test," immersion in water for 30 minutes at 40°C, may be used to monitor sensory recovery

Types
Erb's Palsy

Upper plexus injury to C5 and C6 nerve roots may result in weakness or paralysis in the levator scapulae, rhomboids, deltoid, serratus anterior, supraspinatus, infraspinatus, biceps brachii, brachialis, brachioradialis, forearm supinator, and forearm extensors of the wrist, fingers, and thumb

Klumpke Paralysis/Palsy

Lower plexus injury to C7, C8, and T1 may result in distal weakness or paralysis in the wrist and finger flexors and extensors as well as the intrinsic muscles in the hand

Erb-Klumpke Paralysis/Palsy

Mixed involvement that may include some or all roots from C5 to T1; muscle weakness or paralysis dependent on which roots are included

Limitations

Dependent on the severity and extent of sensory and motor impairment in the involved arm and the presence of associated conditions

Infants may recover from traction injuries spontaneously, whereas recovery from avulsion injuries may be limited; if resolution does not occur within 4 months, prognosis for full recovery is unlikely

Shoulder subluxation and contractures may develop secondary to muscle imbalance according to the following general pattern: glenohumeral adduction and internal rotation, elbow extension, forearm pronation, wrist and finger flexion

HYDROCEPHALUS

Build up in cerebrospinal fluid (CSF) in the brain due to disruption in normal flow of CSF

Most children with spina bifida have hydrocephalus, most often due to Arnold-Chiari malformation, type II

May cause brain damage, resulting in mental retardation due to compression of brain tissue against the skull, seizures, or cranial nerve involvement leading to strabismus, swallowing difficulties, and weak vocal cords

To drain fluid: ventriculoperitoneal shunt (ventricle to peritoneum) or ventriculoatrial shunt (ventricle to atrium of heart)

Signs of shunt malformation

- Irritability
- Vomiting
- Lethargy
- Fever
- Bulging eyes
- Change in behavior, motor coordination, tone, appetite, toileting
- Seizure activity
- Increased muscle tone

SEIZURE DISORDERS

Self-limiting period of unconsciousness, change in behavior, sensation, or autonomic function

Related to change in electrical activity of the brain

Associated with many disabilities with a neurologic basis but can be seen independent of other conditions; approximately 25% of children with developmental disabilities have epilepsy

Epilepsy is a condition of chronic seizures; occurs in approximately 1% of the population

Febrile seizures are isolated and related to a child having a high fever; occur in about 3% of children (Table 2-18)

Epileptic Syndromes
Infantile Spasm (West Syndrome, Infantile Myoclonic Epilepsy)

Begins around 4–8 months of age

Generally occurs in clusters of 4–5 and are jack-knifing jolts with bending forward at the waist

Occurs primarily during periods of drowsiness or when arousing from sleep

Neurodevelopment arrest or regression of skills are common

Common treatment is intramuscular injection of adrenocorticotropic hormone (ACTH)

Lennox-Gastaut Syndrome

Mixed seizure pattern

Often affects children with a history of infantile spasm

Begins between 1 and 8 years of age

Difficult to control with medication

NEUROCUTANEOUS SYNDROME

Genetically based disorders with CNS disturbance and skin abnormalities

TABLE 2-18. Types of Seizures

International Classification	Older Term(s) for Classifying Seizures	Manifestations
Generalized seizure	Generalized seizure	Seizures that are generalized to the entire body; always involve a loss of consciousness; involve entire cortex
Tonic-clonic seizure	Grand mal seizure	Begin with tonic contraction (stiffening) of the body, then clonic movements (jerking) of the body, followed by lethargy or sleep
Tonic seizure Clonic seizure Atonic seizure Absence seizure	Minor motor seizure Drop attacks Petit mal seizure	Stiffening of the entire body; myoclonic jerks start and stop abruptly; sudden lack of muscle tone; nonconvulsive with a loss of consciousness: blinking, staring, or minor movements lasting a few seconds; lack of movement
Akinetic seizure		
Partial seizure	Focal seizure	Seizures not generalized to the entire body; a variety of sensory and/or motor symptoms may accompany this type of seizure

Simple partial seizure
  With motor symptoms
  With sensory symptoms
	Jacksonian seizure	No loss of consciousness or awareness; jerking may begin in one small part of the body and spread to other parts; usually limited to half of the body

Complex partial seizure	Psychomotor seizure Temporal lobe seizure	Sensory aura may precede a motor seizure; Loss of consciousness occurs during the seizure; may develop from a simple partial seizure or develop into a generalized seizure; may include automatisms like lip smacking, staring, or laughing
Unclassified seizure		Seizures that do not fit into the above categories including some neonatal and febrile seizures

Adapted with permission from Ratliffe, K. T. (1998). *Clinical Pediatric Physical Therapy: A Guide for the Physical Therapy Team* (p. 410). St Louis, MO: Mosby.

Tuberous Sclerosis (TS)

Skin abnormalities

- Depigmented white birth marks
- Café au lait spots

CNS abnormalities

- Tubers: large areas of disorganized cortex and white matter
- Associated conditions include glial tumors, hydrocephalus, and retinal tumors
- 90% of individuals with TS develop seizures

Sturge-Weber Syndrome

Congenital port wine stain on face

Venous angiomas (benign blood vessel tumors) associated with CNS abnormalities and progressive cortical atrophy

Aicardi Syndrome
Only seen in girls
Associated with absence of corpus callosum; congenital abnormalities of the eye
Severe mental retardation

HYPOXIC-ISCHEMIC ENCEPHALOPATHY
Asphyxia: hypoxia (lack of oxygen) with ischemia (lack of circulation and acidosis)
Requires resuscitation

Causes
Placental previa
Abruptio placenta
Prolapsed cord
Cephalopelvic disproportion (CPD)
Prolonged labor

Patterns of Abnormalities
Watershed Infarcts
Generalized reduction of cerebral blood flow
Border zone
Severe: results in spastic quadriplegia with mental retardation
Subtle: ADHD, learning disabilities

Focal Infarcts (Strokes)
Major cerebral artery blocked
Usually results in hemiplegia

Diffuse Hypodense Area
Prolonged hypoxia
Multiple cysts or generalized atrophy may develop
Widespread damage: spastic quadriplegia, mental retardation, seizure disorder

Status Marmoratus
Hypoxia to basal ganglia: athetoid cerebral palsy

Prognosis
Correlated with severity of clinical symptoms
Mild neonatal syndrome: no neurologic problems
Severe neonatal syndrome: 75% will die (especially if seizures, coma are present); survivors will have spastic quadriplegia with mental retardation

TRAUMATIC BRAIN INJURY (TBI)
Trauma that results in a change in level of unconsciousness and/or an anatomic abnormality

Causes
Injuries inflicted during accidents (motor vehicle, near drowning, sports and recreation activities), falls, and assaults (gun shot wounds, fights, child abuse)

Types

Depends on force that caused the injury

Impact/contact: scalp injuries, skull fractures, focal brain bruises, epidermal hematomas

Inertial: motion inside the skull creating shear forces; tearing nerve fibers and blood vessels (Box 2-6)

Open head injury: wound that exposes brain to the environment; less common

Closed injury

- Direct injury: Coup–contra-coup
- Shear stresses: most serious

Recovery

Ten stages according to the Rancho Los Amigos Levels of Cognitive Functioning (Malkmus, D., & Stenderup, K. (1974). Rancho Los Amigos, Levels of Cognitive Functioning—Revised. Downey, CA: Rancho Los Amigos Hospital.)

Level I—No response

Level II—Generalized response

Level III—Localized response

Level IV—Confused/agitated: gradual return of cognitive and functional skills

Level V—Confused, inappropriate, nonagitated

Level VI—Confused, appropriate

Level VII—Automatic, appropriate

Level VIII—Purposeful, appropriate: may continue to have difficulties in problem-solving

Level IX—Purposeful, appropriate: may request assistance

Level X—Purposeful, appropriate: may require accomodations

Prognosis

Coma duration: shorter equals a better prognosis

Post traumatic amnesia duration: shorter equals a better prognosis

NEAR DROWNING

Survival at least 24 hours after submersion into fluid

Clinical Features

Hypoxia

Submerged less than 5 minutes—good prognosis

Submerged more than 10 minutes—neurologic impairment

- Coma
- Seizures
- Abnormal posturing, spasticity, rigidity
- Cognitive impairment

BOX 2-6. Types of Traumatic Brain Injuries

Scalp and skull injuries
Brain contusions
Epidural hematomas
Concussions
Diffuse axonal injuries
Acute subdural hematomas

SPINAL CORD INJURY (SCI)

Most common cause is a motor vehicle accident

More likely to sustain cervical injuries

Functional Effects

Table 2-19 shows the functional effects of spinal cord lesions at different levels

Types
American Spinal Injury Association Impairment Scale

Level A: complete injury; no sensory or motor function below S4–5

Level B: incomplete injury; sensory but no motor function below S4–5

Level C: incomplete injury; motor and sensory functioning, but strength less than grade 3

Level D: incomplete injury; strength greater than 3 below the injury

Level E: complete recovery of sensory and motor functioning

Brown-Séquard's Paralysis

Injury to half the spinal cord

Results in hemiplegia

Pain and temperature pathways damaged on opposite side

Anterior Cord

Intact motor function and sensation except proprioception, kinesthesia, vibration; usually caused by partial dislocation or fracture of cervical spine

Sensory disturbance results in inability to walk or control the bowels and bladder

Central Cord Syndrome

Increasing disability in sensory functions, especially pain and temperature

Motor disability greater in upper extremities compared with lower extremities

Stage of Recovery

Stage 1: absence of reflexes, flaccidity, loss of sensation, autonomic dysfunction, spinal shock syndrome (1–6 weeks)

Stage 2: spasticity increases, neurologic return, autonomic dysreflexia

Stage 3: stabilization of loss and recovery of functions

CEREBRAL PALSY (CP)

Persistent lack of postural control and paucity of movement

Due to nonprogressive damage to the CNS before age 3

Prenatal, perinatal, or postnatal in origin

Static encephalopathy that may lead to the development of progressive neuromusculoskeletal limitations

May result from infection, trauma, cranial hypoxia, or consanguinity

Frequently associated with placental insufficiency, prematurity, grade III or IV intraventricular hemorrhage, or periventricular leukomalacia

Diagnosis is difficult during infancy: often diagnosed between 8 and 12 months of age

TABLE 2-19. Functional Effects of Spinal Cord Lesions at Different Levels

Highest Intact Cord Segment	Characteristics	Functional Outcome
C1–3	No voluntary musculoskeletal control below the chin	Comfortable midline seating position, with ventilator tray
C4	Complete respiratory paralysis May have bradycardia, tachycardia, or vomiting Neck movements intact No voluntary function of upper extremities, trunk, or lower extremities Dependent on ventilator support for breathing	Use of "sip and puff" control mechanism for power mobility (chin control possible for C4 injury), environmental control; mouthstick for functional tasks Switch access for computers
C5 Muscles innervated include partial deltoid, biceps, most rotator cuff muscles, diaphragm	Can abduct, extend, and flex shoulder; some flexion of elbow Abdominal respiration as a result of no accessory respiratory muscles; poor respiratory reserve Cannot roll over or get into sitting position without help Abdominal breathing	Adapted joystick mechanism on power wheelchair and environmental control devices Standing pivot transfers with assistance Use of adapted devices for grooming, self-feeding, and accessing computer Older child may be able to perform independent pressure relief through hooking arm and leaning if biceps are strong enough
C6 Muscles innervated include pectoralis major, serratus anterior, latissimus dorsi; complete deltoid and brachioradialis; partial triceps	Good elbow flexion Adduction and internal rotation of shoulder Wrist extension Abdominal breathing	Propels wheelchair using hand rim extensions Independent pressure relief Transfers with assistance and sliding board Assists in dressing and standing pivot transfers Uses universal cuff to write, eat, use computer keyboard
C7 Muscles innervated include triceps, finger flexor and extensor muscles, shoulder depressor muscles	Can lift body weight using shoulder depressors Has weak grasp and release, poor coordination	Independent manual wheelchair propulsion Transfers with minimal assistance Lower extremity with minimal assistance dressing Rolls over, sits up independently
T1–10 Muscles innervated include all upper extremity muscles, trunk muscles above level of injury	Full use of upper extremities Poor trunk balance May use braces for standing	Independent manual wheelchair mobility Drive car or van with hand controls Independent pressure relief

(continued)

TABLE 2-19. Functional Effects of Spinal Cord Lesions at Different Levels (continued)

Highest Intact Cord Segment	Characteristics	Functional Outcome
T10–L2 Muscles innervated include abdominal and upper trunk muscles	Good trunk balance Good respiratory reserve Can accomplish moderate hip-hiking using external oblique and latissimus dorsi muscles	Ambulation with bilateral long leg braces and crutches (energy consuming) Stand or walk functionally in school within small areas Independent wheelchair use
L3 or below Muscles innervated include quadriceps muscle, partial gluteus and hamstring muscles, partial lower extremity muscles depending on level of injury	Poor control of ankles May have lumbar lordosis	Ambulates well, may use short leg braces, walker, crutches or cane, AFO (ankle-foot orthosis) May not use wheelchair May have difficulty getting up from sitting

Adapted with permission from Ratliffe K. T. (1998) *Clinical Pediatric Physical Therapy: A Guide for the Physical Therapy Team* (pp. 288–289). St. Louis, MO: Mosby.

Spastic Cerebral Palsy

Increased muscle tone, typically in antigravity musculature

Muscle imbalance across joints may lead to range of motion limitations of scapular protraction and depression; glenohumeral flexion, abduction, and external rotation; elbow, wrist, and finger extension; forearm supination; hip abduction, extension, and external rotation; knee extension; ankle dorsiflexion; and supination

Spastic Quadriplegia

Involvement of four extremities as well as throat, neck, and trunk musculature

Neonatal feeding dyscoordination and generalized hypotonia may be the first symptoms; if present, low tone gradually transitions to muscle imbalance and spasticity over the first year

Early neuromotor indicators for treatment: very erect head position in prone accompanied by poor ability to flex or right head in supine, elbows flexed and positioned well behind shoulders in prone accompanied by inability to reach or extend hands to midline in supine, little isolated finger motion, extended legs with minimal ankle dorsiflexion

May be associated with seizures; hip subluxation; cognitive, visual, auditory, and oral motor deficits; poor nutrition

Spastic Diplegia

Mainly lower extremity involvement

Gait characterized by short stride length, excessive hip adduction and internal rotation, and ankle plantar flexion

Lower extremity reciprocal movements in crawling and dissociation in all positions difficult to attain

High association with prematurity

Associated with oral motor difficulties, visual deficits, learning disabilities

Spastic Hemiplegia

One side of the body is affected, especially trunk and extremities

Child's tendency is often to disregard affected side and compensate with opposite side

Mild motor milestone delay if present

Equinus deformity secondary to Achilles tendon shortening, a common complication, which can be minimized by early, anticipatory treatment

Increased effort with unaffected side may elicit associated reactions in affected side: upper extremity scapular retraction, shoulder external rotation, elbow flexion, lower extremity adduction, internal rotation, and plantar flexion

May be associated with strabismus; seizures; speech, learning, and perceptual disorders

Ataxic Cerebral Palsy

Generalized decreased muscle tone; infant may initially be diagnosed with "floppy baby syndrome"

Wide base of support (BOS) characteristic in weight-bearing positions

Ataxia and dyscoordination elicited by decreased BOS as the child assumes more erect positions

Hip abduction contractures are occasionally present

May be associated with poor visual tracking and speech delay

High association with abnormal cerebellar development

Athetoid Cerebral Palsy

Extraneous movements associated with postural instability and fluctuating muscle tone, particularly apparent during speech, feeding, and upper extremity activities

High association with maternal-infant Rh incompatibility and hyperbilirubinemia

Cognitive ability typically within normal range

Hearing loss may be present

Mixed Cerebral Palsy

Usually denotes presence of athetosis and spasticity, but may be used to describe other combinations

Other

Rare types of CP that do not correspond to the above categories, including other types of dyskinetic CP or atonic CP, which may be transitional in the young infant and later become spastic or athetoid CP

Prognosis

Walking without aids achieved by children with hemiplegia and some children with diplegia or ataxia; walking with canes, crutches, or Rollator walkers achieved by children with diplegia, some with athetosis, and a few children with quadriplegia

Hypotonia and joint hypermobility with ataxia may decrease with age and increasing level of function

Early Signs and Recognition of Cerebral Palsy

The diagnosis of cerebral palsy may be difficult to definitely make within the first 6 months

Neonatal

Infants at risk because of abnormalities during pregnancy, delivery, or neonatal course

Weak or absent sucking or swallowing

Episodes of bradycardia or apnea

Signs of cerebral irritation such as high-pitched cry or jitteriness

Tone may be decreased

Seizures

Primitive reflexes (e.g., Moro, stepping) may be difficult to elicit

3 Months

Difficulty feeding, tongue thrust may be present

Irritability

Tone usually hypotonic ("floppy baby")

Brisk deep tendon reflexes

Persistent or obligatory primitive reflexes

Child keeps one or both hands fisted

Advanced head control—infant usually has better head control in prone than supine due to extensor tone, but difficulty maintaining head in midline in supine

Strabismus

6 Months

Delayed motor milestones or abnormal patterns (i.e., rolls over by extension of spine instead of segmental rolling)

Preferential unilateral hand use or fisting

Little spontaneous movements; inability to bring hands to midline or reach

Persistence of primitive reflexes

Arching or strong tendency to stand (without sitting)

Infant feels stiff on handling

Difficult to dress

9 Months

Delayed development

Atypical movement

- Crawling: arm movements only; nonreciprocal movements; asymmetrical
- Reaching: splaying of fingers and extended wrist; tremor
- Kicking: nonreciprocal kicking
- Holding arms flexed

12 Months

Scissoring

Toe-walking

Athetoid movements

Handedness

SPINA BIFIDA

Spinal cord and/or vertebrae malformation, usually thoracic or lumbar, as a result of a neural tube defect

Failure of closure of superior neural tube at 3–4 weeks' gestational age results in anencephaly (not compatible with life)

Failure of closure of inferior neural tube at 3–4 weeks gestation results in spina bifida

Increasing evidence for protective role of folic acid against spina bifida; 0.4 mg folic acid per day recommended for women considering pregnancy

Elevated levels of alpha-fetoprotein (AFP) in the prenatal period are a marker for neural tube defects; presence can be determined by ultrasound

Significant risk of hydrocephalus associated with Arnold-Chiari malformation (brainstem and cerebellum herniate through the foramen magnum)

Meningocele

Cyst contains CSF only

Spinal cord remains in appropriate location

Little or no weakness following simple surgical repair

Myelomeningocele (Meningomyelocele or Myelodysplasia)

Cyst contains CSF, and spinal cord is herniated into it

Depending on location and spinal cord extrusion, symptoms range from mild weakness and limited bowel and bladder control to complete paraplegia, associated with hydrocephalus requiring ventriculoperitoneal shunting to drain CSF

Most common type of spina bifida

Myelomeningocele and Hydromyelia

Same as above with addition of central canal greatly distended with CSF

Diastematomyelia

Development of two hemi spinal cords, often separated by a bony spur or block consisting of an incompletely formed vertebrae

May have no neurologic symptoms until growth results in tethered cord and emergence of neurologic sequelae such as rapid onset of scoliosis, lower extremity hypertonus, and urologic symptoms

Tethered cord may occur in association with other types of spina bifida at the original surgical closure site

Spina Bifida Occulta

External appearance of skin over vertebral defect may be normal—tuft of hair, dimple, or sinus leading down to spinal cord

Typically vertebral defect only, nonfusion of vertebral arches

No spinal cord involvement or weakness

Spina Bifida Cystica

External appearance is a fluid-filled cyst

Functional Limitations and Associated Impairments

Decreased mobility and sensation below the level of the lesion

Musculoskeletal deformities including club feet and scoliosis

Cognitive impairments including mental retardation, learning disabilities, and language disorders

Visual impairments

Seizure disorders

Bowel and bladder dysfunction

Skin sores

Latex sensitivity

■ CARDIOPULMONARY

CARDIAC AND ASSOCIATED VESSEL ANOMALIES IN INFANTS AND CHILDREN

Structural cardiovascular anomalies are associated with arrested development occurring during gestational days 18–50

Rubella infection is a documented cause, but maternal drug and alcohol ingestion, radiation exposure, other maternal infections, and maternal diabetes have also been suggested as contributory factors

Significant association with trisomy 21 or Down syndrome

Patent Ductus Arteriosus

Failure of ductus arteriosus to close soon after birth, allowing blood flow from high pressure aorta to pulmonary artery and a left to right shunt

Often associated with prematurity

Typically closed with medication, although surgery may be necessary

Patency of this vessel may be maintained with medication (prostaglandin) to maintain life when more severe anomalies such as hypoplastic left heart syndrome or transposition of great vessels exist

Atrial Septal Defect(s)

Single or multiple openings in the wall separating the two atria, decreasing blood flow going directly to ventricles and resulting in mild to moderate left to right shunt

Patent foramen ovale is the most common atrial septal defect

Often no intervention due to minimal impact on cardiodynamics and eventual closure over time

Ventricular Septal Defect(s)

Single or multiple openings in the wall separating the ventricles, typically resulting in significant left to right shunt and transmission of the high pressures characteristic of the left heart to the pulmonary vascular bed

Pulmonary engorgement results, minimizing the efficiency of oxygenation

Increasing pulmonary vascular resistance over time can create pulmonary hypertension and result in a right to left shunt, followed by cyanosis

Surgical patching is almost always indicated

Coarctation of the Aorta

Narrowing of the aorta in close approximation to the ductus arteriosus

Increased resistance to blood flow in the left ventricle with decreased blood flow to the extremities

Like aortic stenosis, may result in reopening of foramen ovale and creation of a left to right atrial shunt

Surgical correction necessary for resolution

Tetralogy of Fallot

Includes ventricular septal defect, pulmonary stenosis and resulting right ventricular hypertrophy, aortic dextroposition

Significant right to left shunt is the most common cause of cyanosis in children older than 2 years of age

Moderate to severe exercise limitations until surgical correction is completed in stages

Transposition of the Great Vessels

Incomplete division of embryonic exit trunk from heart, resulting in aorta coming from right ventricle, and pulmonary artery from left

Septal defects or patent ductus arteriosus necessary for continued vitality

Cyanosis at rest and severe exercise restriction

Surgical correction in stages

May not lead to reduction or limitations on exercise

Hypoplastic Left Heart Syndrome

Left heart incapable of providing sufficient blood flow to maintain life

Chemical maintenance of patency of ductus arteriosus or creation of atrial septal defect sustains life until heart transplant can occur

Atrioventricular Canal

Atrial and ventricular septa are not fully formed

All four chambers of heart freely communicate

PULMONARY

Asthma

Chronic lung disease with three components

- Reversible airway obstruction
- Airway inflammation
- Increased airway hyperresponsiveness

Characteristics

Bronchial smooth muscle contraction

Mucosa edema, inflammation

Mucus hypersecretion

Males at greater risk

Hispanics and African Americans more at risk than whites

Obesity

Maternal smoking is a risk factors

Classifications

Mild intermittent: symptoms occur less than 2 times per week; asymptomatic between exacerbations

Mild persistent: symptoms greater than 2 times per week may affect activity level

Moderate persistent: daily symptoms; daily inhaler use; exacerbations may affect activity level

Severe persistent: continual symptoms; limited physical activity; frequent exacerbations

■ INTEGUMENTARY

BURNS

Causes

Thermal—primary cause

Electrical

Chemical

Radioactive

Abuse—inflicted

- Approximately 10%
- Usually due to cigarette burns, scalding

Classification

Classification of burns is shown in Table 2–20

Severity

- Size: how much of the body is burned, total percentage of body surface (TPBS)
  - Lund and Browder assessment chart: modified version of "Rule of Nine"
- Severity
  - Classified by American Burn Association
  - Based on type, extent, depth

Stages of Recovery

- Emergent: maintenance of physiologic functioning
- Acute: medically stable; focus on prevention of infection and secondary impairments such as contractures
- Rehabilitative: emphasis on function

■ DEVELOPMENTAL DISABILITIES

A developmental disability is a condition that occurs before age 22, continues indefinitely, is a substantial obstacle to the ability to function, and results in a functional limitation. This definition encompasses some of the disorders previously discussed. However, it also fits conditions such as mental retardation, which can be caused by a variety of etiologies and thus does not fit as neatly under the categories established in the *Guide to Physical Therapy Practice* (1997).

MENTAL RETARDATION

Significantly below average intellectual functioning (Table 2-21)

Onset before 18 years of age (during developmental years)

Adaptive functions are also impaired

Concurrent deficits (communications, self-care, home living, social/interpersonal, use of community resources, self-direction, functional academic skills, work, leisure, health, and safety)

Delay in developmental areas is usually consistent unless associated with another disability such as cerebral palsy

TABLE 2-20. Classifications of Burns

	Partial Thickness			Full Thickness	Full Thickness Plus Underlying Tissue
	Superficial		Deep		
Classification	First degree	First degree	Second degree	Third degree	Fourth degree
Depth of burn	Superficial skin only	Epidermis and a small part of the dermis	Epidermis and a deeper portion of the dermis	All of the epidermis and dermis	Epidermis, dermis and underlying structures of fat, muscle, bone
Appearance	Red, dry; blanches with pressure	Red, blisters, moist; blanches with pressure	Marbled white and red; mottled; blisters	White, brown-black; dry, tough; does not blanch with pressure	White, brown-black; dry, tough; does not blanch with pressure
Sensation	Painful	Very painful	Very painful	No pain or temperature sensation	No pain or temperature sensation
Type of burn	Sunburn, brief scald	Scalds, flash flame	Scalds, flash flame	Flame, contact with hot objects	Flame, contact with hot objects

Reprinted with permission from Ratliffe, K. T. (1998). *Clinical Pediatric Physical Therapy: A Guide for the Physical Therapy Team* (p. 297). St. Louis, MO: Mosby.

TABLE 2-21. Classification of Mental Retardation

Classification	Approximate IQ	Level of Support Needed Throughout Life
Mild	55–70	Intermediate
Moderate	40–55	Limited but consistent
Severe	25–40	Extensive and ongoing
Profound	Below 25	Constant, pervasive

Adapted with permission from Batshaw, M. (1997). *Children with Disabilities* (4th ed., p. 345). Baltimore, MD: Paul H. Brookes.

Prevalence

Approximately 2% of the population

Boys more often than girls (ratio of approximately 2:1)

Associated Disabilities

Mild mental retardation is frequently seen in isolation

Moderate, severe, and profound mental retardation are often seen in conjunction with other impairments such as neuromotor dysfunction, visual impairments, seizures, and behavioral disorders

Causes

It is difficult to determine the etiology of mild mental retardation in children; may be due to genetic and environmental factors

Children requiring extensive support are more likely to have a known biologic etiology

* Most common etiologies are Down syndrome, fragile X syndrome, and FAS
* In general the earlier the biologic insult occurs, the more extensive the level of retardation

SPECTRUM OF PERVASIVE DEVELOPMENTAL DISORDERS (PDD)

Conditions that fall into the spectrum of pervasive developmental disorders are characterized by

* Impairments in social relatedness
* Impairments in communication skills
* Presence of unusual activities (rituals, stereotypes)
* Impairments in sensory motor performance

Prevalence and Causes

Recent indications are that the prevalence is increasing and may be as high as 1 in 500 (Rett syndrome and childhood disintegrative disorder [CDD] are much rarer—1/10,000)

Boys more often affected (3–4:1) (except for Rett syndrome)

Biologic basis includes genetics, metabolic disorders, and neurochemical abnormalities

Conditions on the Spectrum
Autism

Most severe form of PDD

Onset of symptoms often between 18 months and 3 years of age

Communication skills profoundly limited

- Many do not have any communicative skills
- Some may learn to use alternative methods
- Many with verbal language have severely impaired pragmatics
- Receptive language impaired also

Impaired social interactions

- Social recognition: lack of empathy, absence of eye contact
- Social communication: absence of social interaction even as young as 2–3 months; lack of desire to communicate
- Social imagination and understanding: inability to imitate, engage in pretend play, lack of friendship building

Behavioral abnormalities

- Restricted, preservative, and stereotyped behaviors, interests, and activities
- Prefer strict adherence to routines
- Intense attachment to objects or toys
- Restricted use of toys
- Self-stimulating behavior and stereotyped movements
- Decreased attention span
- Mood changes; sleep disturbances; increased sensitivity to noises, touch, or odors; insensitivity to pain and heat

Associated behaviors

- 75% of children also have mental retardation
- Strengths in visual spatial skills and rote memory and weaknesses in language and abstract reasoning

Asperger Disorder

Individuals with behavioral and social challenges seen in autism but not the language and cognitive impairments; often have motor delay and are clumsy

Pervasive Developmental Disorder, Not Otherwise Specified (PDD-NOS)

Neurologically based disorders that can exist with mental retardation, epilepsy, and ADHD

- Abnormal social and communication skills and stereotyped behaviors
- Develop later in childhood
- Not as severe as autism
- It is not uncommon for a child who is eventually diagnosed as having a language-based learning disability to have been initially diagnosed as having PDD-NOS

Rett Syndrome (see page 30)
Childhood Disintegrative Disorder (CDD) or Heller Syndrome

Loss of multiple areas of functioning after at least 2 years of typical development

Behavioral features of autism and mental retardation

LEARNING DISABILITIES

Definition (According to the Individuals with Disabilities Education Act [IDEA] P.L.105-17, 1997)

Disorder in one or more of the basic psychological processes involved in understanding or in using language (spoken or written) and will manifest itself in imperfect ability to listen, think, speak, read, write, spell or do math

Includes perceptual disabilities, dyslexia, aphasia, and dyspraxia

Coexists with other disabilities, most notably ADHD and sensory integrative (SI) dysfunction

Most educational systems require a significant discrepancy between ability and achievement

Associated Impairments

Executive functioning: difficulty using problem-solving strategies; needed or organizational skills, planning, future-oriented behavior, impulse control, vigilance, inhibition

Memory: difficulty in listening, remembering, and repeating auditory stimuli

ATTENTION DEFICIT HYPERACTIVITY DISORDER (ADHD)

Risk Factors

Family history of impulsive, poorly modulated behavior

Prenatal exposure to cocaine, heroin

Preterm birth, low birthweight, neonatal medical complications

Recurring otitis media

Delay in acquisition of language or motor skills

Small head size

Behavioral Red Flags

Poor sleep patterns

Difficult to soothe, modulate behavior

Feeding difficulties

Irritability

Fidgets, difficulty sitting still

Impulsivity

Oppositional

Disruption in parent-child relationship

Can have ADHD without the hyperactivity component

Associated Difficulties

Social skills: difficulties in perceptually based social skills, reading subtle social cues; children tend to be socially isolated

Emotional and behavioral: conduct disorder, withdrawal, poor self-esteem, depression, anxiety, easily frustrated

Motor: difficulties in gross, fine, visual, and perceptual motor skills (see "Sensory Integration" under SI Terminology)

SENSORY INTEGRATIVE (SI) DYSFUNCTION

Sensory integration is the mechanism by which incoming sensations are transmitted, organized, and modulated within the CNS, resulting in an adaptive response

Sensory Systems Involved
Tactile
Discrimination: conscious proprioception, touch pressure, vibration

Protection: detection of damage to the skin

Praxis
The ability to motor plan a new, nonhabitual motor act

Problems: interpreting tactile input, difficulty modulating tactile input

Overregistration (Tactile Defensiveness)
Does the child:

- Seem overly sensitive to rough food textures
- Overdress or underdress
- Avoid using hands or messy play
- Seem to pick fights
- Seem overly sensitive to food or water temperatures
- Seem bothered by clothing tags, seams, types

As a baby did the child:

- Cry excessively
- Have difficulty establishing sleep-wake cycles

Underregistration
Does the child:

- Seem unaware of cuts, bruises
- Mouth objects or clothes excessively
- Touch everything

Both overregistration and underregistration can exist in the same person

Proprioceptive
The understanding of where joints and muscles are in space

Proprioception gives us much information about our body and our movement

Adequate proprioception helps one move smoothly and contributes to praxis

Vestibular
System of balance, equilibrium, movement against gravity

Has been implicated in the development of body posture, muscle tone, ocular-motor control, reflex integration, and equilibrium reactions

Adequate functioning produces the ability to move effectively against gravity

Vestibular problems can result in functional problems of balance and coordination or in modulation problems (underarousal or overarousal) such as gravitational insecurity or intolerance to movement

Signs or Indicators of SI Dysfunction
Overly sensitive to touch, movement, sights, or sounds

Underreactive to sensory stimuli

Activity level that is unusually high or low

Coordination problems (gross and fine motor)

Delays in speech or language skills, motor skills, or academic achievement

Poor organization of behavior

Poor self-concept

SI Terminology

Sensory Integration—process of taking in sensory stimuli and organizing it in the brain. This organization allows the senses to be interconnected, which is necessary for humans to interpret a situation accurately and make an appropriate response.

Adaptive Response—purposeful, goal-directed response to a sensory experience (i.e., a baby sees a rattle and reaches for it).

Sensory Modulation—controls the level of intensity and configuration of incoming sensation and influences our registration of it; balance of inhibition and excitation in the brain.

Sensory Integrative Dysfunction—inability to organize and make sense of incoming stimuli which in turn produces a faulty or disorganized response; there are varying levels of disorder that fall at some point on a continuum.

Sensory Defensiveness—hypersensitive to one or more types of sensation.

Sensory Dormancy—underreactive to sensory input; too much inhibition in the nervous system.

DEVELOPMENTAL DELAY

Failure to achieve developmental milestones as expected based on the typical sequence of development; often associated with hypotonia

Can resolve with remediation but often results in generalized disability such as mental retardation; even with resolution, children are at increased risk for learning disabilities

DEVELOPMENTAL COORDINATION DISORDER

Disorder in movement not associated with a known disability such as cerebral palsy, mental retardation, or a genetic disorder

Associated with learning disabilities, SI dysfunction, ADHD

Children are often poorly coordinated and dyspraxic

Cause is unknown, but CNS inefficiency is suspected

AGING IN PERSONS WITH DEVELOPMENTAL DISABILITIES

It is estimated that more than half a million adults older than 60 years of age have developmental disabilities

Life expectancy and age-related medical conditions are similar to adults in the general population

Individuals with severe cognitive deficits, severe motor impairments, or multiple disabilities have a decreased life expectancy

Higher incidence of Alzheimer's disease in adults with Down syndrome

Higher incidence of osteoporosis and tardive dyskinesia in individuals who have used psychotropic medication for a long time

Higher incidence of obesity in females with mental retardation than seen in the general population

Adults with cerebral palsy note the following musculoskeletal changes: contractures, scoliosis, hip subluxation, dislocation, pathologic fractures, postural pain (often associated with inadequate wheelchair fitting), osteoporosis, and cervical spine stenosis

◼ CANCER

Increasing incidence of cancer in children
Decreasing mortality rates
Uncontrolled proliferation of cancer cells causing various symptomologies
More active than in adults: 80% of children have metastasis

CAUSES

Most unknown
Possible viral link

RISK FACTORS

Exposure to ionizing radiation
Genetic
Pesticides

TYPES

Leukemia

Most common type
Cancer of tissues that make blood cells, including bone marrow and lymph system
Most commonly affects children 2–6 years of age
Sudden or gradual onset
Characteristics include weakness, fatigue, bruising with joint pain

Acute Lymphoid Leukemia (ALL)

Origins in lymph cells
Most common type—affects 80–90% of children with leukemia

Acute Myelogenous Leukemia

Origins in bone marrow
Affects 10–20% of children with leukemia

CNS Cancers

Most common solid tumor
Differentiated by tissue involved and by location (Table 2-22)

Lymphoma
Hodgkin's Disease (HD)

More common in adolescence
More common in boys than girls
Swelling of peripheral lymph nodes with mitosis to bone marrow, spleen, liver, lungs, and
    mediostinum
Prognosis is excellent with early detection and treatment

Non-Hodgkin's Lymphoma (NHL)

More common in young children
More common in boys

TABLE 2-22. Types of Nervous System Tumors in Children

Type of Tumor	Symptoms	Prognosis	Treatment
Astrocytoma Affects almost half of children with brain tumors; two major types			
Cerebellar (about 10–20% of all childhood CNS tumors)	Ataxia, clumsiness, awkward gait, vomiting, headache, irritability, personality changes, fatigue, anorexia	70–90% cure rate	Surgery
Supratentorial (about 35% of all childhood CNS tumors)	Visual disturbances, seizures, headache, vomiting, irritability, personality changes, fatigue, anorexia	75–85% cure rate for low grade, lower for high grade	Surgery; radiation therapy; chemotherapy
Medulloblastoma About 15% of all childhood CNS tumors Usually occurs in the cerebellum	Ataxia, headache, vomiting, irritability, personality changes, fatigue, anorexia	50% cure rate; highest for low grade, lower for high grade	Surgery; radiation therapy
Brain stem glioma About 15% of all childhood CNS tumors	Cranial nerve dysfunction, gait disturbances	Poor	Radiation therapy
Ependymoma (about 5–10% of all childhood CNS tumors)	Seizures, ataxia, clumsiness, hemiparesis, hydrocephalus in infants, headache, vomiting, irritability, personality changes, fatigue, anorexia	50% cure rate	Surgery; radiation therapy
Craniopharyngioma Affects 6–9% of children with CNS tumors	Visual disturbances, headache, vomiting, endocrine disturbances	Benign tumor	Surgery; radiation therapy
Neuroblastoma arises in the sympathetic nervous system with common sites being adrenal glands or paraspinal ganglions; occurs in young children	Pain, abdominal mass, persistent diarrhea, bone pain, pallor, weakness, irritability, anorexia, weight loss	75% for children younger than 1 year of age, 50% for children older than 1 year of age; in some children, the tumor spontaneously regresses	Surgery; chemotherapy; radiation therapy

Reprinted with permission from Ratliffe, K. T. (1998). *Clinical Pediatric Physical Therapy: A Guide for the Physical Therapy Team* (p. 406). St. Louis, MO: Mosby.

Frequently involves abdomen and mediastinum

Prognosis is excellent

Wilms' Tumor (Nephroblastoma)

Genetic with increased incidence in twins and siblings

Tumor of kidney

Associated conditions: microcephaly, mental retardation, growth retardation

Bone Cancers

Soft Tissue Tumors

Most common type: rhabdomyosarcoma or tumor of the striated muscle tissue

Most common in children younger than 5 years of age

Most common sites: head and neck

Fast growing with metastases

Prognosis is excellent (80–90% cure rate) with early identification and vigorous treatment

Measurement

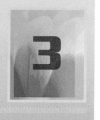

Therapists have long recognized the importance of accurate measurement and information-gathering to determine the needs of children with developmental disabilities, musculoskeletal dysfunction, and other conditions. As in other areas of pediatric physical therapy, there has been an evolution in the types of measurements taken throughout the years. Traditionally, therapists used clinical observations to make intervention decisions. Physical therapists now incorporate a functional outcome approach to determine intervention needs and use standardized tests to determine deviation from age-expected norms. This chapter provides a basic understanding of the measurement process to introduce the reader to a variety of measurement tools and to outline clinical measurement strategies commonly used in pediatric physical therapy.

DEFINITION

The term "measurement" is used in this chapter to encompass the strategies of examination, evaluation, assessment, and screening. Each of these information-gathering strategies has a distinct purpose and will be defined. Generally, the strategies used specifically by physical therapists gather information about an individual's neuromotor, developmental, sensorimotor, musculoskeletal, or cardiopulmonary status.

PURPOSE

Identify risk

Diagnose

Determine eligibility for service

Plan intervention

Document change over time

Determine efficacy of programming

Research

EXAMINATION

According to the American Physical Therapy Association's (APTA) *Guide to Physical Therapist Practice* (1997) (hereafter referred to as *The Guide*), examination is the first element of patient/client management. It is required before any intervention and is performed for all clients. The initial examination has the following three components:

- Patient/client history
- Relevant systems review
- Tests and measures

EVALUATION
The APTA and *The Guide*

An evaluation is a clinical judgment made by a physical therapist based on data gathered from the examination

It reflects the severity of the condition, the possibility of multisystem involvement, the presence of preexisting conditions, and the stability of the condition

Individuals with Disability Education Act (IDEA), Part C, Early Intervention (EI)

An evaluation is conducted to determine developmental status of an infant/toddler, to identify atypical development, to make a diagnosis, and to determine eligibility for early intervention services

An evaluation is done annually

IDEA, Part B, School-Age Services

An evaluation is a process used to determine if a child has a disability

Determines the nature and extent of special education and related services needed by the child

This process is done triannually as requested by the child's multidisciplinary team of service providers (see Chapter 6 for a discussion of eligibility)

ASSESSMENT

The Guide

Measurement or quantification of a variable or the placement of a value on something

IDEA, Part C

Ongoing procedures used for program planning

Determines strengths and needs

Identifies resources, priorities, and concerns of the family

Kirshner and Guyatt (1985)

Define three purposes of assessment

- Evaluative: measures used to determine change over time or change as a result of intervention
- Predictive: measures used to help identify children who will have delays or disabilities in the future or to predict the outcome of the delay or disability
- Discriminative: measures used to distinguish between children who do and do not have a delay, disability, impairment, functional limitation, or atypical development

Approaches to Assessment

Bottom-Up Approach (Fig. 3-1A)

Traditional deficit-driven model

Professional assesses child and determines strengths, needs, and deficit areas; professional determines goals based on findings and determines intervention strategies

Primarily used for identification of disability or delay and/or during the diagnostic process

Useful for identification of impairments

Top-Down Approach (Fig 3-1B)

Outcome-driven model of assessment

Desired outcomes determined first; identify obstacles and strengths of the child and family to obtain outcome; identify strategies to improve performance, bypass obstacles, and reach desired outcome

Ongoing assessment takes place at any point (i.e., identifying obstacles, identifying strengths, and adapting intervention strategies)

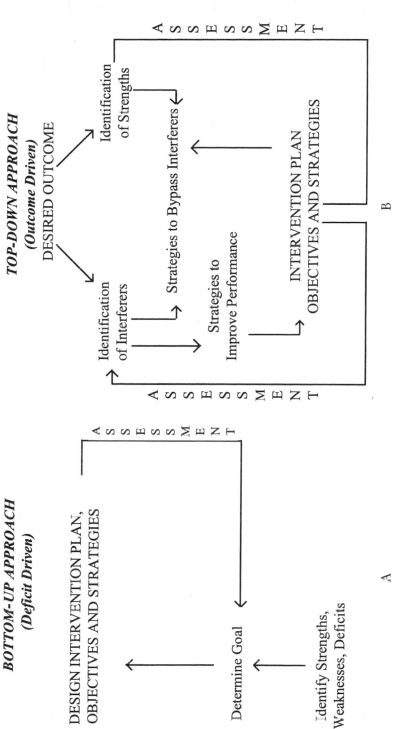

FIGURE 3-1. Two approaches to assessment. **(A)** Bottom-up approach. **(B)** Top-down approach.

Primarily used for program planning

Particularly helpful for children with complex neuromotor and/or cognitive involvement

Routine Based

Identifies those factors, child specific and environmental, that interfere with or promote the performance of a specific functional task within a specific routine

Judges the capabilities of a child within naturally occurring activities and routines

Use of routines promotes the delineation of functional outcomes and intervention strategies

Judgment Based

Completed by parent or caregiver

Enables therapist to obtain task-specific information from individuals who see the child regularly

Yields information that is meaningful to family/caregivers and on what behaviors are considered the typical performance of the child

Ecologic/Naturalistic

Designed to determine a child's ability to perform a functional activity

Takes into consideration the physical, social, and psychological environment in which a task takes place

Provides opportunities for self-initiation, choice, and problem-solving

Places emphasis on adaptive behavior

Yields a description of a child's repertoire across skill domains

Arena Assessment

Simultaneous assessment of the child by various disciplines

Obtains a holistic, integrated view of the child's skills across domains

Reduces handling of the child by multiple examiners and redundant questioning of caregivers

Team designs a format before the assessment which is based on individual needs of the child and family

Used primarily for program planning of a child identified as having a developmental delay or disability

Assessment Standards

Any procedure or strategy used to gather information about a child should adhere to four standards (Box 3-1)

SCREENING

APTA, The Guide

Screenings are done to determine the need for:

• Primary, secondary, or tertiary prevention services

• Further examination, intervention, or consultation

• Referral to another health care practitioner

IDEA

Screenings are done as part of "Child Find" to locate those children at risk for a developmental delay, disability, or functional limitation as defined under Parts C and B

BOX 3-1. Assessment Standards

Treatment Validity

Does the assessment identify feasible goals and objectives for the child and family?

Does assessment information assist in the selection or use of intervention methods or approaches?

Does the assessment contribute to evaluating intervention effects?

Social Validity

Does the assessment identify goals and objectives that are judged as worthwhile and appropriate to the family, caregivers, or society?

Are assessment methods and materials acceptable to the participants?

Does the assessment detect social significance of change?

Convergent Validity

Are several types of assessment materials and approaches used?

Is information collected from several settings and sources, especially family members?

Are assessments done on more than one occasion?

Consensual Validity

Is information pooled and perspectives shared?

Do team dynamics favor collaboration and negotiation?

Are decisions truly consensual?

■ METHODS USED TO MEASURE OR GATHER INFORMATION

Parental/caregiver questionnaires and/or interviews

Naturalistic observations

Clinical observations

Direct testing

USE OF STANDARDIZED TESTS

Information gathered is usually child-centered

Examiner adheres to specific instructions, administration, and scoring of each item

Tests should possess sound psychometric characteristics

Findings often result in a standard score or developmental age

Requires training to administer test and interpret findings

Can be norm-referenced or criterion-referenced (Table 3-1)

Psychometric Characteristics of Standardized Tests
Validity

The degree to which a meaningful interpretation can be inferred from a measurement

Content

How well the items of an instrument represent the theoretical basis of the trait to be measured

TABLE 3-1. Standardized Measurement Instruments	
Norm-Referenced	**Criterion-Referenced**
Standard point scores	Cut-off scores
Compares individual performance against group performance	Compares performance against described criteria
Normal distribution of scores desired	Variability of scores not obtained, mastery of skills desired
Maximizes differences among individuals	Discriminates between successive performances of one individual
Requires diagnostic skills of examiner	Provides information to plan therapy/instruction
Not sensitive to effects of therapy or instruction	Sensitive to effects of intervention
Not concerned with task analysis	Depends on task analysis
Summative	Formative

Adapted with permission from Cook, D. G. (1991). The assessment process. In W. Dunn (Ed.), *Pediatric Occupational Therapy: Facilitating Effective Service Delivery.* Thorofare, NJ: Slack Inc.

Construct
How well the instrument as a whole accurately represents the theoretical basis of the trait to be measured

Criterion-related
How well the instrument correlates with another instrument purporting to measure the same construct or trait

Concurrent
How well two instruments that claim to measure a specific trait and are administered simultaneously correlate with one another

Predictive
How well one instrument given at one time correlates with another instrument purporting to measure same trait administered at a later time

Reliability

The degree to which an instrument produces consistent/repeatable results

Internal Consistency
The degree to which all items of the test are measuring the same concept

Interrater
Degree of agreement between two or more testers of the same test given to the same individual (percent agreement, intraclass correlation coefficient [ICC], Kappa)

Standard Error of Measurement
Used to develop a range of probable scores around the obtained score that is likely to indicate the child's "true" ability level on that test

Test-Retest
Correlation between two administrations of the same test to the same individual on two separate occasions

Accuracy
Sensitivity
Ability of the instrument to detect dysfunction/abnormality (positive finding)

Specificity
Ability of the instrument to detect normality (negative finding)

Scores
Provide information on how a child performs in comparison to other children or specific criteria

Standard Scores (Fig 3-2)
Compares the scores received by one child to the scores received on the same test by a specific population of children

Based on the normal distribution of scores

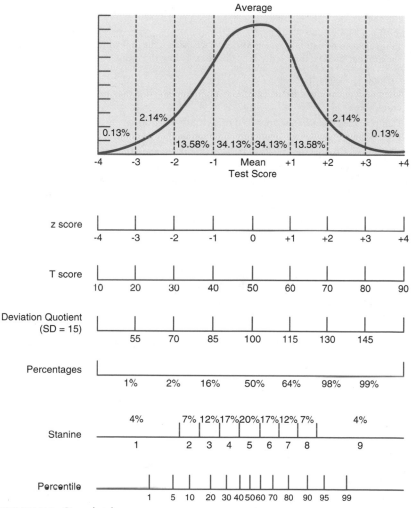

FIGURE 3-2. Standard scores.

Precise method to compare the score of one child with his or her peers

Deviation or developmental quotient

- Allows for comparability of scores across ages
- Norm-referenced
- Normally distributed
- The mean is typically 100 with an SD of 15

Percentile ranks

- Ranking based on the percentage of individuals in the normative sample who received a score above or below the score received

Stanine (standard nine)

- Single-digit score (1–9) based on mean and SD of the group

T score

- Equivalent to a deviation quotient and Z score, although mean is 50 with an SD of 10

Z score

- Equivalent to deviation quotient and T score using a mean 0 with an SD of 1; indicates the number of SD units a score falls above or below the mean

Age/Grade Equivalent Score

- Used to determine at what age an "average" child receives the raw score received by the child tested
- Can provide an inaccurate appraisal of a child's performance

Standardized Tests Used by Pediatric Physical Therapists

The following section contains descriptions of a wide variety of tests that can be used by pediatric physical therapists. The tests are arranged in alphabetical order. To assist the reader, the tests have been divided by age and if they are norm- or criterion-referenced in Table 3–2. Some instruments span age groups, and some are used with only a portion of children within an age group. For example, the AIMS is used for children up to 18 months of age only.

AGES & STAGES QUESTIONNAIRE REVISED (ASQ)
Diane Bricker, Jane Squires, and Linda Mounts

PURPOSE
To determine the developmental level of a child through parent report

AGE RANGE
4–60 months

AREAS TESTED
Communication
Gross motor
Fine motor
Problem-solving
Personal-social

(continued)

(*continued*)

PSYCHOMETRIC CHARACTERISTICS

Norm referenced, standardized on 2008 children primarily from Oregon

Internal consistency: Cronbach's Alpha across subtests = 0.53 in gross motor at 4 months to 0.87 in gross motor at 12 and 16 months; correlation between domain score and overall score: Pearson r = 0.54 in gross motor at 16 months, 0.83 in personal-social at 12 months, problem-solving at 30 months, and problem-solving at 36 months

Test-retest reliability: percent agreement at 2-week intervals: 94% (SEM, 0.10)

Interrater reliability: percent agreement between parent and professional: 94% (SEM, 0.12)

Concurrent validity: with a variety of standardized instruments at various ages ranged from 67% between the ASQ and Standford-Binet at 24 months to 100% with the McCarthy Scales at 30 months and 36 months, most over 80%

Sensitivity: 75% overall, range = 51% (4 months) to 90% (36 months)

Specificity: 86% overall, range = 81% (16 months) to 92% (36 months)

ADMINISTRATION

Parents complete the questionnaire. Program staff convert each response to a point score, total the score, and compare the total to established cut-off points.

TIME REQUIRED

15–30 minutes to administer and 5 minutes to score

ADVANTAGES

- Cost-effective monitoring system
- Strong psychometric characteristics
- Encourages family collaboration
- Provides a mechanism to consider the typical performance of the child in addition to the performance seen during a formal professionally administered assessment
- Can be used in conjunction with home visits or within a primary medical care clinic
- Items are written in simple language at the 4th- to 6th-grade reading level
- Decreases need for frequent clinic visits
- Companion videotape describing use of the ASQ on home visits
- Spanish version available
- Instructions for scoring questionnaires with incomplete data

LIMITATIONS

- Subjectivity of parent and examiner
- Cut-off scores cannot be used for children falling outside the 2-month age range for each questionnaire
- Screening tool only

ORDERING INFORMATION

Paul H. Brookes Publishing Co.
PO Box 10624
Baltimore, MD 21285-0624

TABLE 3-2. Tests Categorized by Age

Birth–3 Years	3–5 Years	5 Years and Older
Alberta Infant Motor Scale (AIMS)*	Ages and Stages Questionnaire (ASQ)	Developmental Test of Visual Motor Integration (VMI)*
Assessment, Evaluation and Programming System for Infants and Children (AEPS)	Developmental Test of Visual-Motor Integration (VMI)*	Battelle Developmental Inventory (BDI)*
Assessment of Preterm Infant Behavior (APIB)	Battelle Developmental Inventory (BDI)*	Battelle Developmental Inventory – Screen (BDI-S)*
Ages and Stages Questionnaire (ASQ)	Battelle Developmental Inventory – Screen (BDI-S)*	Brigance Diagnostic Inventory of Early Development (BDIED-R)
Battelle Developmental Inventory (BDI)*	Brigance Diagnostic Inventory of Early Development (BDIED-R)	Bruininks-Oseretsky Test of Motor Proficiency (BOTMP)*
Brigance Inventory of Early Development – Revised (BDIED-R)	Bayley Scales of Infant Development – Second Edition (BSID-II)*	Clinical Observations of Motor and Postural Skills (COMPS)
Bayley Infant Neurodevelopmental Screener (BINS)*	Bruininks-Oseretsky Test of Motor Proficiency (BOTMP)*	Denver Developmental Screening Test – Second Edition (DDST-II)*
Bayley Scales of Infant Development – Second Edition (BSID-II)*	Denver Developmental Screening Test – Second Edition (DDST-II)*	Developmental Test of Visual Perception (DTVP)*
Carolina Curriculum for Infants and Toddlers with Special Needs – Second Edition (CCITSN)	Developmental Programming for Infants and Young Children (DPIYC)	FirstSTEP Screening Test for Evaluating Preschoolers (FIRST STEP)*
Denver Developmental Screening Test-II (DDST)*	Developmental Test of Visual Perception (DTVP)*	Functional Outcome Assessment Grid (FOAG)
Developmental Programming for Infants and Young Children (DPIYC)	FirstSTEP: Screening Test for Evaluation Preschoolers (FIRSTSTEP)*	Gross Motor Function Measure (GMFM)
Erhardt Developmental Prehension Assessment (EDPA)	Functional Outcome Assessment Grid (FOAG)	Motor Free Visual Perceptual Test – Revised (MFVPT-R)*
Functional Outcome Assessment Grid (FOAG)	Gross Motor Function Measure (GMFM)	Movement Assessment Battery for Children (Movement ABC)*
Gross Motor Function Measure (GMFM)	Miller Assessment of Preschoolers (MAP)	Peabody Developmental Motor Scales-2 (PDMS)*
Hawaii Early Learning Profile (HELP)	Motor Free Visual Perceptual Test – Revised (MFVPT-R)*	Pediatric Evaluation of Disability Inventory (PEDI)*
Infant Toddler Developmental Assessment – Provence Profile (IDA)	Movement Assessment Battery for Children (Movement-ABC)	Scales of Independent Behavior – Revised (SIB-R)*
Infant Developmental Screening Scale (IDSS)	Peabody Developmental Motor Scales-2 (PDMS)*	School Function Assessment (SFA)
		Sensory Integration and Praxis Test (SIPT)

(continued)

TABLE 3-2. Tests Categorized by Age (Continued)

Birth–3 Years	3–5 Years	5 Years and Older
Infant Motor Screen (IMS)	Pediatric Evaluation of Disability Inventory (PEDI)*	Sensorimotor Performance Analysis (SPA)
Infant Neurological International Battery (INFANIB)	Scales of Independent Behavior – Revised (SIB-R)	Sensory Profile
Infant Toddler Symptom Checklist (ITS)	Sensory Integration and Praxis Test (SIPT)	Test of Gross Motor Development-2 (TGMD)*
Movement Assessment of Infants (MAI)	Test of Gross Motor Development – 2 (TGMD)*	Test of Visual Motor Integration (TVMI)*
Milani-Comparetti Motor Development Screening Test (MCMDST)	DeGangi-Berk Test of Sensory Integration (TSI)	Test of Visual Perceptual Skills – Non Motor (TVPS-NM)*
Meade Movement Checklist (MMCL)	Test of Visual Motor Skills (TVMS)*	Transdisciplinary Play Based Assessment (TPBA)
Neonatal Individualized Developmental Care, Assessment and Programming (NIDCAP)	Test of Visual Motor Integration (TVMI)*	Functional Independence Measure for Children (Wee-FIM)
Neonatal Behavioral Assessment Scale – Second Edition (NBAS)	Test of Visual Perceptual Skills – Non Motor (TVPS-NM)*	Vulpe Assessment Battery – Revised (VAB-R)
Neonatal Oral-Motor Assessment Scale (NOMAS)	Toddler and Infant Motor Evaluation (TIME)*	
Neonatal Neurobehavioral Examination (NNE)	Transdisciplinary Play Based Assessment (TPBA)	
Neurological Assessment of the Preterm and Full-Term New Born Infant (NAPFI)	Functional Independence Measure for Children (Wee-FIM)	
Neurological Exam of the Full Term Infant (NEFTI)	Vulpe Assessment Battery – Revised (VAB-R)	
Peabody Developmental Motor Scales-2 (PDMS)*		
Pediatric Evaluation Disability Inventory (PEDI)*		
Scales of Independent Behavior-Revised (SIB-R)*		
Test of Sensory Function in Infants (TSFI)		
Test of Visual Motor Skills (TVMS)*		
Toddler and Infant Motor Evaluation (TIME)*		

CHAPTER 3

(continued)

TABLE 3-2. Tests Categorized by Age (Continued)		
Birth–3 Years	**3–5 Years**	**5 Years and Older**
Transdisciplinary Play Based Assessment (TPBA)		
Functional Independence Measure for Children (Wee-FIM)		
Vulpe Assessment Battery – Revised (VAB-R)		

These tests are norm referenced.

ALBERTA INFANT MOTOR SCALE (AIMS)

Martha C. Piper and Johanna Darrah

PURPOSE

To identify infants and toddlers with gross motor delay and to evaluate gross motor skill maturation over time

AGE RANGE

Birth–18 months

AREAS TESTED

Fifty-eight gross motor skill items divided among four positions: prone, supine, sitting, and standing

Each item observed for weight-bearing, posture, antigravity movement

PSYCHOMETRIC CHARACTERISTICS

Standardized on more than 2000 children

Interrater reliability: Pearson r = 0.95–0.00

Test-retest reliability: Pearson r 5 0.86–20.99

Concurrent validity with PDMS, Pearson r = 0.90–0.99, (typically developing children) and 0.84–0.98 (abnormal and at-risk)

Discriminant validity: Pearson r = 0.89

ADMINISTRATION

Observation of spontaneous movement of infant in four positions. Minimal handling is required and parents are encouraged to be the primary facilitator. Descriptions in manual specify criteria of weight-bearing, posture, and antigravity movement.

TIME REQUIRED

20–30 minutes (can take as little as 10–15 minutes)

ADVANTAGES

- Sound psychometric qualities
- Observation only
- Can be used in well-baby clinics
- Minimal equipment needed
- Manual provides exceptional diagrams and photographs of each item

(continued)

(continued)

LIMITATIONS

- Standardized on Canadian children; thus, the sample may not reflect the same demographic variables of the U.S. population
- Limited age range
- Cannot be used with older children with disabilities

ORDERING INFORMATION

WB Saunders Company
The Curtis Center
Independence Square West
Philadelphia, PA 19106

ASSESSMENT, EVALUATION, AND PROGRAMMING SYSTEM FOR INFANTS AND CHILDREN (AEPS), VOLUME 1: MEASUREMENT FOR BIRTH TO THREE YEARS; VOLUME 2: THREE TO SIX YEARS

Diane Bricker

PURPOSE

To determine level of skill attainment; assist in the development of programmatic outcomes, goals, and objectives; and monitor progress toward attainment of outcomes over time

AGE RANGE

Developmental skill range from 1 to 36 months of age or 3 to 6 years

AREAS TESTED

Fine motor

Gross motor

Adaptive

Cognitive

Social

Communication

Psychometric Characteristics of Volume 1

Criterion referenced

Interrater reliably: Pearson $r = 0.70$ (social domain) to 0.96 (gross motor domain, total test score)

Test-retest reliably: Pearson $r = 0.77$ (social domain) to 0.95 (gross motor, total test)

Concurrent validity with BSID: MDI $r = 0.93$, PDI $r = 0.88$; Gesell $r = 0.51$

ADMINISTRATION

Individually administered or observed within the context of naturally occurring events. A three-point scoring system is used. Qualifying notes are also coded indicating if an item was scored by observation, direct testing, or reporting and if an item was performed with adaptations or modifications

(continued)

(continued)

ADVANTAGES

- Links measurements to specific curriculum; items are related to program goals, objectives
- Allows for observation or direct testing
- Takes into consideration modifications or adaptations to the task
- Administered during naturally occurring events
- Variety of forms provided that encourage family and team participation
- Data recording forms, curriculum, family report measure, family interest survey, and child progress chart included
- Companion volumes for assessing children 3–6 years of age and 2 curriculums (one for each age group, i.e., 0–3 and 3–6)

LIMITATIONS

- Administered across domains and environments, may make data collection time-consuming
- Does not provide normative information, standard scores, nor age equivalents
- Encourages team participation in data collection which may be cumbersome initially
- Motor sections limited and may be inappropriate for children with severe disabilities
- Familiarity with activity-based approach to early intervention is helpful

ORDERING INFORMATION

Paul H. Brookes Publishing Co.
PO Box 10624
Baltimore, MD 21285-0624

ASSESSMENT OF PRETERM INFANT BEHAVIOR (APIB)

Heidelise Als, Barry Lester, Edward Z. Tronick, and T. Berry Brazelton

PURPOSE

To describe the behavioral organization and repertoire of the preterm infant and to document behavioral change over time

AGE RANGE

Medically stable infants who were born preterm and infants born full-term

AREAS TESTED

Based on the synactive theory of development, the APIB assesses five subsystems of behavior:

- Physiologic/autonomic
- Motor organization
- State organization
- Attentional/interactive
- Self-regulatory

PSYCHOMETRIC CHARACTERISTICS

Interrater reliability: percent agreement = 0.90 with training

Predictive validity of the APIB to various tasks measuring neuropsychological processing at 5 years of age: Kendall tau = 0.52. Marked differences (Kendall

(continued)

(continued)

tau = 0.83) between preterm and full-term infants on autonomic, motor, attentional, and interactive dimensions

ADMINISTRATION

Examiner presents six graded sequences of increasingly demanding environmental inputs. Records stress and self-regulation behaviors into three groups: autonomic, motoric, and state-related. Scoring procedures vary according to package and yield three scores for each system (baseline, reaction, postmaneuver), yielding 283 mutually exclusive scores that can be reduced to 30 summary variables. There are three additional score sheets. Six summary scores identify differential subsystem stability of the infant; the others quantify specific functions.

TIME REQUIRED

Can take up to 3 hours to administer and score

ADVANTAGES

- Provides information on the infant's reaction to environmental changes
- Appropriate, developmental intervention to reduce stress and optimize the infant's behavioral organization and abilities can be developed from findings
- Appropriate for use in research

LIMITATIONS

- Requires extensive training for administration and interpretation
- Lengthy to administer
- Not feasible for routine clinical use
- Can use tool only if infant is medically stable, in an open crib, and breathing room air

ORDERING INFORMATION

Heidalise Als
Children's Hospital
320 Longwood Avenue
Boston, MA 02115

BATTELLE DEVELOPMENTAL INVENTORY (BDI)
Jean Newborg, Joh Stock, Linda Wnek, John Guidubaldi, and John Svinicki

PURPOSE

To determine developmental level of infants and young children, plan intervention strategies, and assess effects of instruction

AGE RANGE

Birth to 8 years

AREAS TESTED

Personal-social
Adaptive
Motor

(continued)

(*continued*)

Communication

Cognition

PSYCHOMETRIC CHARACTERISTICS

Norm referenced, standardized on 800 children divided among 10 age groups

Standard error of measurement for domain scores: range = 0.32 for adaptive domain at 6–11 months to 9.05 for total score at 48–59 months

Test-retest reliability: Pearson r = −0.99 for total sample; 0.84 (cognitive domain at 12–17 months) to 0.99 (total score at 6–11, 12–17, 24–35, and 36–47 months; adaptive domain at 6–11, 12–17, and 18–23 months; personal-social at 12–17 and 18–23 months; and motor at 6–11 months)

Concurrent validity with Vineland and Developmental Activities Screening Inventory strong for total test score (0.94 and 0.91, respectively) and subdomain scores (0.78–0.93); correlation low to moderate with full scale WISC-R (0.42–0.79) and Standford-Binet (0.41–0.61); with PEDI: 0.73; not significant with BSID MDI (−0.03, total score; −0.02 to −0.15 domain scores)

ADMINISTRATION

Administered through structured format, interviews with caregivers, and/or naturalistic observations. Three-point scoring system. Raw scores are converted to percentiles, standard scores, and age equivalents.

TIME REQUIRED

Less than 1 hour for children younger than 3 years of age or older than 5; 1.5–2 hours for children between 3 and 5 years of age

ADVANTAGES

- Companion screening test containing 96 of 341 test items
- Guidelines provided for administering items to children with disabilities
- Blends criterion-referenced with norm-referenced features
- Covers all developmental areas
- Subdomain scoring can indicate strengths and needs
- Items can be scored by parent report
- Instructional activities available
- Computerized scoring program available

LIMITATIONS

- Concurrent validity studies done with very small samples
- Each subdomain contains very few items and may not represent the full developmental sequence
- Test materials must be purchased and come in large cardboard box that is difficult to transport in addition to a box with test manuals and examiner's manual
- Standard scores for infants are based on a very small sample size
- Age-related discontinuities in summary scores have been noted to affect eligibility significantly

ORDERING INFORMATION

Riverside Publishing Company
8420 Bryn Mawr Avenue
Chicago, IL 60631

BATTELLE DEVELOPMENTAL INVENTORY SCREENING TEST (BDI-S)

Jean Newborg, John R. Stock, and Linda Wnek

PURPOSE

Screening test derived from the Battelle Developmental Inventory to determine if a comprehensive evaluation is necessary

AGE RANGE

Birth to 8 years

AREAS TESTED

Personal-social

Adaptive

Motor

Communication

Cognitive

PSYCHOMETRIC CHARACTERISTICS

Norm-referenced, standardized on 800 children divided among 10 age groups

Specific reliability studies were not performed using only the screening test; as items are derived from the full BDI, one could assume that reliability would be similar

Validity determined on a sample of 164 children from the norming and clinical populations

Correlation for total test and between the BDI and the screening test were all above 0.90

ADMINISTRATION

Same as BDI.

TIME REQUIRED

10–30 minutes

ADVANTAGES

- Guidelines provided for administering items to children with disabilities
- Covers all developmental areas
- Items can be scored by parent report
- Cut-off scores based on standard deviations and probabilities

LIMITATIONS

- Reliability studies not conducted specifically for screening test
- Test materials come in a large cardboard box that is difficult to transport in addition to a box with test manuals and examiner's manual
- The screening test is part of full BDI; cannot be purchased separately

ORDERING INFORMATION

Riverside Publishing Company

8420 Bryn Mawr Avenue

Chicago, IL 60631

CHAPTER 3

BAYLEY INFANT NEURODEVELOPMENTAL SCREENER (BINS)

Glen P. Aylward

PURPOSE

To identify infants who are at risk for delays or neurologic impairments

AGE RANGE

3–24 months

AREAS TESTED

Items are categorized into four "conceptual areas of ability":

- Basic neurologic functions/intactness
- Receptive functions: visual, auditory, verbal
- Expressive functions: gross motor, fine motor, vocalizations
- Cognitive processes

PSYCHOMETRIC CHARACTERISTICS

Norm-referenced, standardized on a sample of 600 nonclinical infants

Clinical validity sample included 303 infants who had low birthweights, were small for gestational age, were born prematurely, and had medical complications

Internal consistency: Cronbach's Alpha = 0.73 (3 months, 12 months) – 0.85 (24 months)

Test-retest reliability (nonclinical sample only): Pearson r = 0.71 (3 months), 0.83 (9 months, 0.84 (18 months)

Decision consistency: percent agreement for classification = 72% (3 months), 68% (9 months), and 78% (18 months)

Interrater reliability (nonclinical sample only): Pearson r = 0.79 (6 months), 0.91 (12 months), 0.96 (18 months)

Classification agreement with BSID-II: varies depending on age range but generally higher agreement between low-risk classification on BINS and WNL classification on BSID-II; with BDI: excellent percent agreement occurs between low risk on BINS and normally developing on BDI

Concurrent validity with BSID-II 5 0.39 (6 months, PDI) to 0.82 (24 months, MDI); Pearson r with BDI 5 0.16 (18 months, motor) to 0.51 (12 months, cognitive)

Correct classification: 54–80% of nonclinical sample, 62–89% of clinical sample

ADMINISTRATION

Standardized procedures. Administered by an experienced examiner. Incorporates some items from the BSID-II in addition to muscle tone and movement quality, but is not a mini-BSID-II. Administration and scoring has been modified. Guidelines are given in accepting parental report.

TIME REQUIRED

10 minutes

ADVANTAGES

- Incorporates neurologic items with developmental items
- Standardized on both clinical and nonclinical samples
- Incorporates items and administration procedures from the BSID-II

- Time-efficient
- Requires only a few materials that are contained in a kit, but can use child's own toys if necessary to engage infant
- Indicates on scoring sheet which conceptual area an item is testing
- Training video available
- Manual provides information on performance of items by children with various medical complications

LIMITATIONS

- Validity is low to moderate
- Reliability moderate for nonclinical sample
- Requires the constructing or purchasing of a set of steps for which dimensions are given
- Caregiver reporting can be used only on a limited number of items
- Criteria of many items, especially muscle tone, are not clear

ORDERING INFORMATION

Psychological Corporation
19500 Bulverde Road
San Antonio, TX 78259

BAYLEY SCALES OF INFANT DEVELOPMENT-II

Nancy Bayley

PURPOSE

To identify developmental delay and to monitor a child's developmental progress

AGE RANGE

1 to 42 months

AREAS TESTED

Mental: language, perceptual
Motor: gross, fine
Behavior

PSYCHOMETRIC CHARACTERISTICS

Norm referenced

Interrater reliability: Pearson r = 0.75 (motor scale, PDI), 0.96 (mental scale, MDI)

Test-retest reliability: Pearson r = 0.78 (motor scale, PDI), 0.87 (mental scale, MDI)

Concurrent validity with McCarthy Scales of Children's Abilities: Pearson r = MDI: 0.57–0.77; PDI: 0.18–0.59; with WPPSI-R MDI: 0.21–0.73: PDI: 0.14–0.41); additional studies also indicate that the BSID-II, mental scale correlates better with other tests that assess general cognitive ability. Motor scale correlates moderately with motor subtests of general developmental examinations such as the McCarthy. Correlations of the motor scale to other developmental scales indicate that the motor scale measures constructs relatively independent of the constructs in general developmental tests

(*continued*)

(continued)

ADMINISTRATION

Individually administered test using standardized materials, instructions, and criteria. Items arranged according to degree of difficulty. Binary scoring system (pass/fail).

TIME REQUIRED

25–60 minutes to administer and score, depending on child's age and tolerance for test

ADVANTAGES

- Most widely used tool to determine developmental level of infants
- Most widely used assessment in infant research
- Sound psychometric properties
- Standardized on a large and nationally representative sample

LIMITATIONS

- No subscores available to quantify specific strengths and needs
- Binary scoring systems does not allow for credit for emerging skills
- Cognitive items rely on fine motor response
- Limited assessment of quality of movement
- Reliability for the motor scale is moderate only
- Validity of motor scale to other motor tests not established

ORDERING INFORMATION

Psychological Corporation
19500 Bulverde Road
San Antonio, TX 78259

THE BEERY-BUKTENICA DEVELOPMENTAL TEST OF VISUAL-MOTOR INTEGRATION — 4TH EDITION, REVISED WITH SUPPLEMENTAL DEVELOPMENTAL TESTS OF VISUAL PERCEPTION AND MOTOR CONTROL

Keith E. Beery

PURPOSE

To help identify significant difficulties that some children have in integrating or coordinating their visual perceptual and motor abilities

AGE RANGE

3–18 years of age

AREAS TESTED

Visual-motor integration

Visual perception

Motor coordination

PSYCHOMETRIC CHARACTERISTICS

Internal consistency: Alpha: 0.82 for VMI, 0.81 for visual, 0.82 for motor

Interrater reliability: 0.94 for VMI, 0.98 for visual, 0.95 for motor

Test-retest reliability at 3-week intervals: 0.87 for VMI, 0.84 for visual, 0.83 for motor

(continued)

(continued)

Concurrent validity with a variety of standardized instruments at various ages ranged from 52% between the VMI and WRAVMA Drawing subtest to 75% with the Copying subtest of the DTVP-2. Low correlations exist between the VMI and the Bender Gestalt, with ranges from 29–93% with a moderate median of 56%. The Visual Perception supplemental test was correlated with the DEVP-2 Position in Space at 62% and the Motor Coordination supplemental test with the DTVP-2 Eye Hand Coordination at 65%.

Predictive validity: 85% of kindergarten children scoring low on the VMI and 3 other shorter tests were identified as having reading problems 7 years later

ADMINISTRATION

There are three parts to the VMI. On the Visual Perception Test, the child matches shapes by pointing. On the Motor Coordination Test, the child traces within boundaries with a pencil. On the Visual-Motor Integration Test, the child copies shapes with a pencil. There is specific scoring criteria for each item and part. The raw scores are computed and converted to standard scores, percentiles, and age equivalents.

TIME REQUIRED

10–15 minutes

ADVANTAGES

- No special equipment necessary to administer
- Relatively inexpensive to administer and score
- Easy to administer and score
- Well researched
- Provides suggestions for teaching visual-motor integration
- Differentiates which aspect contributes to visual-motor integration difficulties, visual perceptual difficulties and/or motor coordination difficulties
- May be useful in assessment of perceptual-motor readiness for successful handwriting production for typically developing kindergartners

LIMITATIONS

- Limited in types of tasks required (i.e., on the VMI subtest the child is only required to copy geometric designs)

ORDERING INFORMATION

Modern Curriculum Press
Simon and Schuster
299 Jefferson Road
PO Box 480
Parsippany, NJ 07054-0480

BEHAVIORAL CHARACTERISTICS PROGRESSION (BCP)

VORT Corporation

PURPOSE

Curriculum-based assessment to identify areas of need in an individual's behaviors

AGE RANGE

1–14 years developmental age

(continued)

(continued)

AREAS TESTED

Cognition

Language

Gross motor

Fine motor

Social

Self-help

Vocational

PSYCHOMETRIC CHARACTERISTICS

Criterion-referenced

ADMINISTRATION

Individually administered in collaboration with family members or caregivers. Information is collected by direct observation during daily activities and play, structured elicited situations, and parent interview. The team chooses which behavioral strands may be areas of priority. Scores are transferred onto a simple profile sheet to display the individual's overall progress and development.

TIME REQUIRED

Can be administered over time

ADVANTAGES

- Encourages a multidisciplinary approach
- Provides an instructional activities booklet to complement the assessment
- Designed to be used with specific curriculum intervention strategies
- Requires no verbal directions
- Families are encouraged to make choices and preferences in all aspects of assessment and planning

LIMITATIONS

- Does not provide standardized scores
- Little research to establish efficacy or psychometric information

ORDERING INFORMATION

VORT Corporation
PO Box 60132
Palo Alto, CA 94306

BRIGANCE INVENTORY OF EARLY DEVELOPMENT, REVISED EDITION (BDIED-R)

Albert H. Brigance

PURPOSE

To determine a developmental level and to assist in program planning

AGE RANGE

Birth–7 years

(continued)

(continued)

AREAS TESTED

Psychomotor

Self-help

Speech and language

General knowledge and comprehension

Early academic skills

Social-emotional

PSYCHOMETRIC CHARACTERISTICS

Criterion-referenced; items were chosen from a variety of norm-referenced tests

No psychometric information reported

Field tested in 43 school systems across 16 states

ADMINISTRATION

Begin at the developmental level determined to be most appropriate for a given child. The skills that a child demonstrates within the skill sequence are circled in the developmental record book. The record book also has a bar graph that can be colored to provide a visual representation of the child's performance. Age range for accomplishment of each item is in the record book.

TIME REQUIRED

Varies depending on age level, skill of child, and method used; can be given over time

ADVANTAGES

• Useful for program planning

• Administration procedures are flexible

• Does not require specialized materials

• Variety of methods allowed: parent interview, observation, formal and informal procedures

• Provides references for the sequencing and grouping of items

• Additional materials include resources for parents and professionals, tools for developing individual education programs (IEPs), and a tracking system

• Is compatible with Brigance Prescriptive Readiness

LIMITATIONS

• Does not consistently consider qualitative aspects of performance

• Lacks psychometric information

• Most effective for use with children with mild to moderate disabilities

ORDERING INFORMATION

Curriculum Associates

5 Esquire Road

North Billerica, MA 01862-2589

BRUININKS OSERETSKY TEST OF MOTOR PROFICIENCY (BOTMP)
Robert H. Bruininks

PURPOSE

To assess motor skills of individual children and develop and evaluate motor training programs

(continued)

(*continued*)

AGE RANGE

4.5–14.5 years

AREAS TESTED

Running speed and agility

Balance

Bilateral coordination

Strength

Upper-limb coordination

Response speed

Visual-motor control

Upper-limb speed and dexterity

PSYCHOMETRIC CHARACTERISTICS

Norm-referenced, standardized on 765 children divided among 10 age groups

Interrater reliability: visual motor control subtest: Pearson r = 0.63 (copying a circle with preferred hand) to 0.97 (cutting out a circle with preferred hand, drawing a line through a path with preferred hand)

Test-retest reliability: Pearson r at grade 2 = 0.77 for gross motor composite, 0.88 for fine motor composite, 0.89 for battery composite; Pearson r at grade 6 = 0.85 for gross motor composite, 0.68 for fine motor composite, 0.86 for battery composite. Short form: 0.87 for grade 2 and 0.84 for grade 6.

Subtest test-retest reliability range from 0.29 (upper limb coordination at grade 6) to 0.89 (upper limb speed and dexterity at grade 2 and strength at grade 6)

Standard error of measurement: 2.0 (upper limb speed and dexterity) to 4.7 (fine motor composite)

Validity differentiates between typically developing children and those with mental retardation and learning disabilities

Construct validity: relationship between subtest scores and chronologic age 0.78

ADMINISTRATION

Individually administered test using standardized testing equipment and instructions. Contains a short form, a modified version of the complete battery, that can be used as a screen.

TIME REQUIRED

45–60 minutes for complete battery;15–20 minutes for the short form

ADVANTAGES

- Standardized kit available with all necessary equipment
- Includes a short form that is useful for screening
- Interesting and different testing items
- Norm-referenced motor test with standard scores available for children older than 10 years of age

LIMITATIONS

- May be difficult to administer to younger children because of significant length
- Instructions are complicated and may be difficult for children with mental retardation or language disorders/delays/disabilities

(*continued*)

(continued)

- All items must be administered although earlier failures may indicate that a child cannot accomplish more advanced tasks; may not be good for children who are easily frustrated by failure
- Standardized scores based on 1970 census; thus, information may be outdated
- Test-retest reliability of individual subtests weak
- Limited research on its characteristics and appropriateness for use with various populations

ORDERING INFORMATION

American Guidance Service
Publisher's Building
PO Box 99
Circle Pines, MN 55014–1796

CANADIAN OCCUPATIONAL PERFORMANCE MEASURE (COMP)

Mary Law, Sue Baptiste, Anne Carswell, Mary Ann McColl, Helene Polatajko, and Nancy Pollock

PURPOSE

To detect change in client's or family's perception of occupational performance over time

AGE RANGE

All ages

AREAS TESTED

Self-care

Productivity

Leisure

PSYCHOMETRIC CHARACTERISTICS

Interconsistency reliability: Pearson r = 0.41–0.56 for performance, 0.71 for satisfaction

Test-retest reliability: ICC 0.63 for performance score, 0.84 for satisfaction

Responsiveness: significant change scores ($p < 0.0001$) between first assessment and reassment with a variety of clients

ADMINISTRATION

Client or family chooses up to five problematic tasks and rates each of these using a 10-point scale on performance and satisfaction on completing each task A total satisfaction and performance score are calculated. The changes in performance and satisfaction over time are calculated for each problem to indicate progress.

TIME REQUIRED

30–40 minutes, on average

ADVANTAGES

- Easy to administer
- Can be used with all age groups and all disabilities
- No equipment needed
- Client is a partner in rehabilitation

(continued)

(*continued*)

- Helps therapist to implement a client-centered, functional approach
- May be helpful to engage older child or adolescent in own programming

LIMITATIONS

- Some clients have difficulty with the rating scale
- Some clients may have difficulty with identifying the problems for intervention, particularly in the early stages of disability
- Can be difficult for clients with cognitive impairments

ORDERING INFORMATION

CTTC Building, Suite 3400
1125 Colonel By Drive
Ottawa, Ontario K1S5RI

THE CAROLINA CURRICULUM FOR INFANTS AND TODDLERS WITH SPECIAL NEEDS, 2ND EDITION (CCITSN)

Nancy M. Johnson-Martin, Kenneth G. Jens, Susan M. Attermeier, and Bonnie J. Hacker

PURPOSE

Curriculum-based assessment used to determine approximate developmental level of children and programming strategies

AGE RANGE

Birth–24-month developmental range

AREAS TESTED

Cognition
Communication
Social/adaptation
Fine motor
Gross motor

PSYCHOMETRIC CHARACTERISTICS

Criterion-referenced

Interrater reliability (1st edition): percent agreement: 97%

Field-tested in 22 intervention programs in North Carolina and in 10 national sites for efficacy: results indicated that children made progress in the sequences that were the focus of intervention

ADMINISTRATION

Individually administered or in collaboration with parent or caregiver. Parent report is accepted. The items are sequenced in order of expected development.

TIME REQUIRED

Varies, can be administered over time

ADVANTAGES

- Developed for use with children with disabilities
- Contains a large representative sample of items for each domain

(*continued*)

(continued)

• Includes instructions for integrating interventions into child's daily routines, including adaptations for disability
• Designed to be used with specific curricular intervention strategies
• Places emphasis on adaptive functional skills

LIMITATIONS
• Does not provide standardized scores
• Little research to establish efficacy or psychometric information

ORDERING INFORMATION
Paul H. Brookes Publishing Co.
PO Box 10624
Baltimore, MD 21285-0624

CAROLINA CURRICULUM FOR PRESCHOOLERS WITH SPECIAL NEEDS (CCPSN)

Nancy M. Johnson-Martin, Susan M. Attermeier, and Bonnie J. Hacker

PURPOSE
Curriculum-based assessment used to determine approximate developmental level of children and programming strategies

AGE RANGE
2–5 years developmental range

AREAS TESTED
Cognition
Communication
Social adaptation
Fine motor
Gross motor

PSYCHOMETRIC CHARACTERISTICS
Criterion-referenced
No established reliability

ADMINISTRATION
Individually administered or in collaboration with parent or caregiver. Interventionists fill in the assessment log by observing the child and beginning each sequence at the level where the child has accomplished many skills but not all the skills. The items are scored as pass, fail, or emerging. A developmental progress chart is completed, revealing a profile of skills. Teaching activities can be found in the assessment log.

TIME REQUIRED
Can be administered over time

ADVANTAGES
• No specific materials or kit
• Covers all developmental areas

(continued)

(*continued*)
- Links assessment to specific curriculum
- Provides suggestions on adapting intervention strategies for children with special needs
- Administered during naturally occurring events
- Assessment log may be completed over several days or weeks
- Supplies information for goals and objectives of the IEP

LIMITATIONS
- Lacks research to establish validity and reliability
- Does not result in a standardized score; therefore, must be used in conjunction with a standardized test if standardized scores are required for eligibility purposes

ORDERING INFORMATION
Paul H. Brookes Publishing Co.
PO Box 10624
Baltimore, MD 21285-0624

CHOOSING OPTIONS AND ACCOMMODATIONS FOR CHILDREN (COACH)
Michael F. Giangreco, Chigee J. Cloninger, and Virginia S. Iverson

PURPOSE
To identify a child's educational outcomes and instructional strategies based on family priorities and team decision-making

AGE RANGE
Students aged 3–21 years identified as having moderate to profound disability

AREAS TESTED
Cross-Environmental
- Communication
- Socialization
- Personal management
- Leisure and recreation
- Applied academics

Environment-Specific
- Home
- School
- Community
- Vocational

PSYCHOMETRIC CHARACTERISTICS
Criterion-referenced
No established validity and reliability

ADMINISTRATION
After an evaluation that determines eligibility for services, a student planning team is formed and performance in the above areas is determined to develop a program plan.

(*continued*)

(continued)

TIME REQUIRED

60–90 minutes for each part

ADVANTAGES

- Outlines valued life outcomes that are meant to provide a balance between independence and interdependence with others
- Based on inclusion of the family in all aspects of an individual's educational program
- Motor, cognitive, and sensory areas are embedded in all cross-environmental and environment-specific activities, allowing for discipline-free goals to be developed
- Emphasizes problem-solving methods to improve effectiveness of educational planning
- A self-monitoring and peer-coaching guide is provided to increase user proficiency
- Is helpful for prioritizing and cross-prioritizing goals among disciplines
- Requires team to value inclusion, collaboration, and transdisciplinary practice

LIMITATIONS

- Does not result in a standard score; therefore, must be used in conjunction with standardized test if standardized scores are required for eligibility purposes
- No research to establish validity and reliability

ORDERING INFORMATION

Paul H. Brookes Publishing Co.
PO Box 10624
Baltimore, MD 21285-0624

CLINICAL OBSERVATIONS OF MOTOR AND POSTURAL SKILLS (COMPS)

Brenda N. Wilson, Nancy Pollack, Bonnie Kaplan, and Mary Law

PURPOSE

To screen children for subtle motor coordination problems

AGE RANGE

5–9 years

AREAS TESTED

Slow movements

Arm rotation

Finger-nose touching

Prone extension posture

Asymmetrical tonic neck reflex

Supine flexion posture

PSYCHOMETRIC CHARACTERISTICS

Test-retest reliability: ICC for children with developmental coordination disorders (DCD), 0.87; for children without DCD, 0.76; total, 0.93

Interrater reliability: ICC = 0.57 (between occupational therapists with pediatric experience and those without, with children with DCD) to 0.88 (between occupational therapists with pediatric experience with total sample of children)

(continued)

(continued)

Internal consistency: Cronbach's Alpha: 0.77 for total score

Discriminant validity: total test score discriminates children with DCD from those without

Concurrent validity: Pearson r = 0.40 with motor accuracy test-revised, 0.48 with VMI, 0.46 with standing balance, eyes open

Sensitivity: 100% for 5 year olds and 8–9 year olds, 82% for 6–7 year olds

Specificity: 63–90%

ADMINISTRATION

Individually administered as outlined in the manual. Scoring varies with each item.

TIME REQUIRED

15–20 minutes

ADVANTAGES

- Procedures simple and straightforward, only equipment needed is the elbow measurement tool that comes with the manual
- May be helpful for treatment planning
- Manual provides information on relation of item to underlying sensory-motor substrate

LIMITATIONS

- Screening tool only
- Sample size to calculate cut-off points very small (n = 36); thus, results must be interpreted with caution

ORDERING INFORMATION

Therapy Skill Builders
19500 Bulverde Road
San Antonio, TX 78259

DEGANGI-BERK TEST OF SENSORY INTEGRATION (TSI)

Georgia A. DeGangi and Ronald A. Berk

PURPOSE

To screen for sensory integrative dysfunction in preschool children

AGE RANGE

3–5 years

AREAS TESTED

Postural control

Bilateral motor integration

Reflex integration

PSYCHOMETRIC CHARACTERISTICS

Criterion-referenced

Pilot studies to establish construct validity performed on 101 typically developing children and 38 children with known delays

Interrater reliability: ICC = 0.15 (reflex integration) to 0.82 (postural control)

(continued)

(continued)

Test-retest reliability: Pearson r = 0.85 (postural control) to 0.95 (total test score)

Decision consistency: po = 0.79 (reflex integration) to 0.93 (bilateral motor integration, total test score)

Discriminative reliability: 79% of items discriminated between typically developing children and those with sensory processing dysfunction

Sensitivity: 0.66 (reflex integration) to 0.84 (bilateral motor integration)

Specificity: 0.64 (bilateral motor integration) to 0.85 (total test)

Classification accuracy: 0.81 for total test score

ADMINISTRATION

Items administered in order presented in the manual. Multipoint scoring system reflecting the degree to which a skill has been developed. Total point scores are calculated and compared with a profile of scores corresponding to three levels (normal, at risk, and deficient) in two age groups (3–4 years and 5 years).

TIME REQUIRED

30 minutes

ADVANTAGES

- A screen for vestibular-based functions of sensory integration
- Most testing materials come in testing kit
- Provides practitioners with a validated rating scale for sensory integrative dysfunction in preschoolers rather than relying on clinical observations

LIMITATIONS

- Does not provide standardized scores
- Construct validity established with a small number of children with a known delay, and sample was not representative of the population
- Designed as a screening device and needs to be combined with other test results for diagnostic purposes
- Subtests primarily assess vestibular-based functions and not full domain of sensory integration
- Few children in the 5-year age range were included in the initial test development studies; thus, it may not be appropriate for older preschool-aged children

ORDERING INFORMATION

Western Psychological Services
12031 Wilshire Boulevard
Los Angeles, CA 90025

DENVER-II

William K. Frankenburg, Josiah Dodds, Phillip Archer, Beverly Bresnick, Patrick Maschka, Norman Edelman, and Howard Shapiro

PURPOSE

To detect potential developmental problems in young children and monitor children who are at risk for developmental problems

AGE RANGE

1 week–6 years, 6 months of age

(continued)

(continued)

AREAS TESTED

Personal-social: behavior, caring for self

Fine motor-adaptive: eye-hand coordination, manipulation of small objects, problem-solving

Language: hearing, speaking, understanding

Gross motor: sitting, walking, jumping

Also, five subjective "test behavior" items assessing overall test behavior

PSYCHOMETRIC CHARACTERISTICS

Norm-referenced, standardization on a nonclinical sample of 2096 children in Colorado

Interrater reliability: percent agreement = 0.99 (0.95–1.00); Kappa 0.75

Test-retest reliability: percent agreement = 0.90 (0.50–1.00); Kappa 0.75 for 59% of items, Kappa 0.40 for 23% of items

Sensitivity: 0.83

Specificity: 0.43

ADMINISTRATION

Individually administered using materials supplied in the kit. Standardized administration procedures are described in the manual, with key criteria and procedures on the back of the test form. The total score is based on the numbers of items passed or failed in relation to the age of the child. The score is categorized as normal, suspect, or untestable. "Test behaviors" are completed after administration of the test.

TIME REQUIRED

15 minutes

ADVANTAGES

- Training videotape available
- Training sessions held twice yearly
- Details on initiating a community screening program contained in the technical manual
- Technical manual also provides suggestions for conducting a training program
- Companion Denver Developmental Activities available
- Companion prescreening developmental questionnaire (PDQ) is completed by parents

LIMITATIONS

- Sample based on children living in Colorado only; thus, may not be representative of the overall population of children
- Although reliability strong, no other psychometric characteristics reported

ORDERING INFORMATION

Denver Developmental Materials, Inc.
PO Box 6919
Denver, CO 80206-0919

DEVELOPMENTAL PROGRAMMING FOR INFANTS AND YOUNG CHILDREN—REVISED (DPIYC)

D. Sue Schafer, Martha S. Moersch, and Diane B. D'Eugenio

PURPOSE

To describe the developmental status of a child with a disability and assist with program planning and implementation

(continued)

(continued)

AGE RANGE

Early Intervention Developmental Profile (EIDP): 0–36 months

Preschool Developmental Profile (PDP): 36–60 months

AREAS TESTED

Cognition

Gross motor

Fine motor

Language

Social-emotional

Self-care

PSYCHOMETRIC CHARACTERISTICS

Criterion-referenced

Interrater reliablity of EIDP: percent agreement = 0.89

Test-retest: Pearson r = 0.93–0.97 at 3-month intervals, 0.90–0.97 at 6-month intervals

Concurrent valildity of EIDP with BSID MDI: r = 0.80–0.96; with BSID PDI: r = 0.62–0.95; with Vineland Social Maturity Scale: 0.77–0.93; with REEL: 0.33–0.75

Concurrent validity of EIDP of gross motor subtests with PDMS, gross motor scale: r = 0.85; of fine motor subtests with PDMS, fine motor scale: r = 0.79

No psychometric properties reported on PDP

ADMINISTRATION

A five-volume set. Developmental checklist individually administered by any member of a multidisciplinary team in the home, clinic, school, or early intervention setting. Materials are not provided, but a list of the needed materials is provided. Highest passed item in each subtest is marked in the profile graph, arranged by developmental levels. Profile is used to indicate strengths and weaknesses. No numeric score is obtained.

TIME REQUIRED

1 hour

ADVANTAGES

• Can be used in early intervention through preschool

• Contains stimulation activities and behavioral objectives linked to test items

• Can be used by a variety of team members

• Gross motor sections contain items related to the integration of primitive reflexes and the development of automatic reactions

• Each domain was developed by disciplinary specialists

LIMITATIONS

• Few items in each category

• Little research to determine effectiveness in accurately describing behavior in children with disabilities

• Operational definitions of test items allow subjective interpretations

• Large number of test materials need to be gathered by examiners

ORDERING INFORMATION

University of Michigan Press

389 Greene Street

Ann Arbor, MI 48104

CHAPTER 3

DEVELOPMENTAL TEST OF VISUAL PERCEPTION—2ND EDITION (DTVP-II)

Donald D. Hammil, Nils A. Pearson, and Judith K. Voress

PURPOSE

To determine visual perceptual and visual motor abilities

AGE RANGE

4–10 years of age

AREAS TESTED

Form constancy

Figure ground

Position in space

Spatial relation

PSYCHOMETRIC CHARACTERISTICS

Norm-referenced

Internal consistency: Cronbach's Alpha: 0.80–0.97 for subtests, 0.93 or above for composite

Interrater reliability: >0.92 for subtests, 0.98 for total test

Test-retest reliability: 0.80–0.92 for subtests, 0.95 for total test

SEM: 2–3 for composite scores

Discriminant validity: discriminates between children with and without learning disabilities

Concurrent validity: with the MVPT: 0.89 for motor items only, 0.87 for total test; with the VMI: 0.72 for nonmotor items only, 0.78 for total test

ADMINISTRATION

The child is asked to point to one of several choices of pictures or use a pencil to trace, copy, connect dots, or make marks. Subtest raw scores are converted into age equivalents, percentiles, and standard scores. Composite scores are also obtained for motor reduced visual perception and visual-motor integration as well as general visual perception. These composite scores are converted to quotients, percentiles, and age equivalents.

TIME REQUIRED

30–60 minutes

ADVANTAGES

• Distinguishes between visual perception and visual motor problems

• Computerized scoring program is available

LIMITATIONS

• More research is needed on the relationship between the DTVP-II and cognitive abilities

• Reliability associated with subtests is generally near or below the level of acceptability; thus, not as accurate as composite scores

ORDERING INFORMATION

PRO-ED, Inc.

8700 Shoal Creek Boulevard

Austin, TX 78757

ERHARDT DEVELOPMENTAL PREHENSION ASSESSMENT (EDPA)—2ND EDITION

Rhonda P. Erhardt

PURPOSE

To describe the quality of prehension patterns for treatment planning

AGE RANGE

Birth–15 months

AREAS TESTED

Positional-reflexive: involuntary arm-hand patterns

Cognitively directed: voluntary movements of approach, grasp, manipulation, and release

Prewriting skills: pencil grasp and drawing

PSYCHOMETRIC CHARACTERISTICS

Criterion-referenced

Interrater reliability: ICC: 0.42–0.85, percent agreement: 65–90%, Spearman rank order correlation: median of 0.77 with a range of 0.54–0.91 (right) and a median of 0.77 with a range of 0.54–0.96 (left)

Intrarater reliability: Spearman rank order correlation: median 0.91 (right), 0.88 (left)

Construct validity: EDPA and PDMS, FM 0.95 (right), 0.94 (left), EDPA and chronologic age 0.95 (both hands)

Concurrent validity: significantly different age equivalent scores found between EDPA and PDMS, FM

ADMINISTRATION

Administered or observed items using readily available materials. Scored using a descriptive procedure indicating well established, emerging or abnormal pattern, not present, or transitional pattern. Done bilaterally as appropriate.

TIME REQUIRED

Not specified; varies according to experience of examiner

ADVANTAGES

- Examples of treatment planning provided
- Separate scores for each hand, for comparison
- Provides reproducable score sheets
- Items are pictorially presented
- Items arranged in developmentally sequenced clusters
- Videotapes are available that discuss development of hand function
- Screening form available for individuals 15 months of age through adulthood

LIMITATIONS

- Detailed information on administration and scoring of pattern components is not provided
- Unable to calculate standard scores
- No testing material provided
- Lacks test-retest reliability

(continued)

CHAPTER 3

(continued)
ORDERING INFORMATION
Therapy Skill Builders
19500 Bulverde Road
San Antonio, TX 78259

FIRSTSTEP: SCREENING TEST FOR EVALUATING PRESCHOOLERS (FIRSTEP)

Lucy Jane Miller

PURPOSE

To identify young children who are at risk for mild to severe school-related problems

AGE RANGE

2 years, 9 months–6 years, 2 months

AREAS TESTED

Cognition

Communication

Motor

Social-emotional

Adaptive behavior

Parent/teacher scale

PSYCHOMETRIC CHARACTERISTICS

Norm-referenced, standardization sample: 1433 children divided among 7 age groupings

Internal consistency: averaged across age groups = 0.71(motor) to 0.92 (social-emotional)

Interrater reliability: percent agreement of scaled scores = 0.88 (motor) to 0.96 (language, cognitive); of classification = 0.81 (social-emotional) to 1.00 (language)

Standard error of measurement: 0.67 (social-emotional at 2:9–3:2 years) to 3.68 (composite score at 3:3–3:8 years)

Test-retest reliability: percent agreement = 0.82 (social-emotional) to 0.91 (language)

Concurrent validity: composite score with MAP total test r = 0.71; with WPPSI-R total test r = 0.82; with BOTMP battery composite r = 0.63

Sensitivity: 74% (motor) to 85% (cognitive)

Specificity: 81% (motor) to 82% (cognitive)

ADMINISTRATION

Individually administered following standardized procedures, most of which come in the kit. Each subtest contains four "games," each having one or more items specific to each of the seven age groups. Scoring procedures are specific to each item. Raw scores are converted to domain scores, which can be converted to scaled scores or composite scores. Composite scores are interpreted as within acceptable limits, below acceptable limits and warranting further assessment, or slightly below acceptable limits and warranting further monitoring before referral for comprehensive evaluation.

(continued)

(continued)

TIME REQUIRED

15 minutes

ADVANTAGES

- Covers all developmental areas
- Strong standardization and psychometric properties
- Items fun for children
- Score sheets provide visual aids to add in efficiency of administration
- Training video available
- Spanish version available

LIMITATIONS

- Most test materials come in the kit, but the examiner must provide others
- Some believe it may have cultural bias
- Takes longer than 15 minutes
- Some motor items require specific set-up procedures affecting efficiency of administration

ORDERING INFORMATION

The Psychological Corporation
19500 Bulverde Road
San Antonio, TX 78259

FUNCTIONAL OUTCOMES ASSESSMENT GRID (FOAG)
Phillipa H. Campbell

PURPOSE

To assist the team in developing and implementing functional outcomes for children with disabilities

AGE RANGE

No specific age range

Individualized based on desired outcomes; thus, age is not a factor

AREAS TESTED

Caring for self

Communication

Learning and problem-solving

Mobility

Play and leisure skills

Socialization

Performance areas and performance components delineated within each outcome area

Based on the American Occupational Therapy Association's document, "Uniform Terminology for Occupational Therapy, 2nd edition"

PSYCHOMETRIC INFORMATION

No psychometric information reported

(continued)

(continued)

ADMINISTRATION

Individualized observation of functional skill performance to determine which components (physical, environmental, behavioral, sensory) are affecting positively or negatively the child's performance of a skill. Each component is scored on a five-point scale from no problems to significant problem that affects or prevents skill performance.

TIME REQUIRED

Varies depending on the child and number of tasks assessed

ADVANTAGES

- Directly links assessment to program planning
- Based on team desired outcomes
- Operationalizes top-down assessment strategy
- Individualized to meet unique needs of a child
- Facilitates integrated service provision

LIMITATIONS

- Lacks psychometric data
- No aggregate score
- Cannot be used to determine skill acquisition level, diagnosis, or eligibility

ORDERING INFORMATION

Campbell, P. H., & Forsyth, S. (1993). Integrated programming and movement disabilities. In M. Sneel (Ed.), *Instruction of Students with Severe Disabilities* (4th ed., pp. 751–811). Columbus: Merrill.

GROSS MOTOR FUNCTION MEASURE (GMFM)

Dianne Russell, Peter Rosenbaum, Carolyn Gowland, Susan Hardy, Mary Lane, Nancy Plews, Heather McGavin, David Cadman, and Sheila Jarvis

PURPOSE

To evaluate change in gross motor function in children with cerebral palsy, describe a child's current level of motor function, and determine treatment goals

AGE RANGE

No specific age range is recommended by the authors; however, the test has been validated on children between 5 months and 16 years

Seems best suited for children 2–5 years

AREAS TESTED

Lying and rolling

Sitting

Crawling

Standing

Walking, running, and jumping

PSYCHOMETRIC CHARACTERISTICS

Criterion-referenced

Interrater reliability: ICC = 0.75 (lying and rolling) to 0.97 (standing)

(continued)

(continued)

Intrarater reliability: ICC = 0.75 (lying and rolling) to 0.99 (all other subtests and total score)

Percent agreement: 96.2–98.4

ADMINISTRATION

Individually administered with a demonstration and three trials for each item. Specific scoring criteria for each item based on a four-point Likert scale measuring how much of the item the child completes. Dimension scores and a total score are obtained. Each dimension score and the total score are converted to a percentage of the maximum score for that dimension.

TIME REQUIRED

45–60 minutes

ADVANTAGES

• Specifically designed for children with cerebral palsy
• Concerned with quantity of movement, not quality
• Measures change over time

LIMITATIONS

• No normative data
• Directions regarding support with arms not clear
• Many items scored based on length of movement or time maintenance in a position, etc., which may not be reflective of functional aspect of skills
• General scoring key is based on how much of the item the child accomplishes (initiates, <10%, etc.); however, most items are scored based on specific criteria

ORDERING INFORMATION

Chedoke-McMaster Hospitals
Chedoke Campus, Building 74
Box 2000, Station A Hamilton
Ontario, Canada, L8N 3Z5

CHAPTER 3

INFANT MOTOR SCREEN (IMS)

Robert E. Nickel

PURPOSE

To determine the neuromotor status of infants born prematurely

AGE RANGE

4–16 months corrected age

AREAS TESTED

Muscle tone

Primitive reflexes

Automatic responses

Symmetry

PSYCHOMETRIC CHARACTERISTICS

Criterion-referenced

Interrater reliability: 0.81 0.90 for individual items, 0.91–1.00 for total test rating

(continued)

(*continued*)

Sensitivity at 4 months to detect cerebral palsy: 0.93; at 8 months: 1.0

Specificity at 4 months to detect cerebral palsy: 0.89; at 8 months: 0.96

ADMINISTRATION

Test items are administered in a specific sequence. Items are scored separately for each side of the body. If the scores differ, the highest score is used for total score classification. Scores classified into normal, suspect, or abnormal for corrected age.

TIME REQUIRED

15 minutes or less

ADVANTAGES

- Instructions are clear
- Line drawings on test form facilitate scoring
- Reliability strong
- Quantifies neurologic findings
- Specifically designed to be used with infants born prematurely
- Limited literature based on its uses

LIMITATIONS

- Sreening tool only
- Because it was designed to be used with children born prematurely, it may not be sensitive enough to be used with lower-risk infants
- Sensitivity/specificity data for 4- and 8-month-old children only

ORDERING INFORMATION

Child Development and Rehabilitation Center
The Oregon Health Sciences University
Clinical Services Building
Eugene, OR 87043

INFANT/TODDLER SYMPTOM CHECKLIST: A SCREENING TOOL FOR PARENTS (ITS)

Georgia A. DeGangi, Susan Poisson, Ruth Z. Sickel, and Andrea Santman Wiener

PURPOSE

To identify infants at risk for sensory integrative disorders, attentional deficits, and emotional or behavioral problems

AGE RANGE

7–30 months

AREAS TESTED

Five age-specific checklists (7–9, 10–12, 13–18, 19–24, and 25–30 months) containing information on

- Self-regulation
- Attention
- Eating or feeding
- Dressing, bathing, touch

(*continued*)

(continued)

- Movement
- Listening and language
- Looking and sight
- Attachment/emotional functioning

There is also a general screening version

PSYCHOMETRIC CHARACTERISTICS

Criterion-referenced

Construct validity: medium to large discrimination index reflecting differences in item performance

Decision validity: false delayed rate: 3% (19–24 months) to 13% (25–30 months); false normal rate: zero (19–24 months) to 14% (25–30 months)

Concurrent validity: few intercorrelations between the ITS Checklists and the TSFI, Test of Attention in Infants (TAI), and the BSID-II, Mental Scale

ADMINISTRATION

Six checklists (five are age-specific, and one is a general screen). Completed by the parent or used by a professional as part of a parent interview. Used alone as a screen or can be used as a part of comprehensive diagnostic evaluation. Raw scores for each category (never/sometimes, most times, or past) are summed. Compare total score to checklist cut-off scores to determine normal or deficient category.

TIME REQUIRED

10 minutes

ADVANTAGES

- Provides information that is distinct from that obtained by other measures
- Can be used as a parent report tool or as part of an interview
- Uses family-friendly terms
- Quick
- Provides structure for clinical and parental observations and concerns

LIMITATIONS

- Psychometric properties are limited
- Screening test only; should not be used alone for diagnosing sensory processing dysfunction

ORDERING INFORMATION

Therapy Skill Builders
19500 Bulverde Road
San Antonio, TX 78259

INFANT-TODDLER DEVELOPMENTAL ASSESSMENT (IDA)—PROVENCE PROFILE

Sally Provence, Joanna Erikson, Susan Vater, and Saro Palmeri

PURPOSE

To determine a performance age range and a descriptive summary of developmental competencies

(continued)

(continued)

AGE RANGE

Birth–3 years

AREAS TESTED

Gross motor

Fine motor

Relationship to inanimate objects

Language/communication

Self-help

Feelings, social adaptation, and personality traits

PSYCHOMETRIC CHARACTERISTICS

Criterion-referenced

Interitem consistency: Alpha = 0.77 (self-help) to 0.96 (language)

Intrerrater reliability: percent agreement among three practitioners with nine children = 81% for language/communication to 91–95% for other domains

Concurrent validity: compared percentage of children classified as "delayed" on three tools (BSID, Vineland, and Provence Profile); Provence Profile and Vineland identified similiar percentage of children

Predictive validity: determined by follow-up survey to 15 community agencies to which IDA referrals were made; 83% of the 12 agencies responding indicated that referrals were appropriate

ADMINISTRATION

Administered by interdisciplinary team of two or more professionals and parents using standardized procedures, play-based observation, and parental reports in an arena format. Test materials are included in the kit. Items totaled to determine a performance age that can be transformed into a percent delay.

TIME REQUIRED

Varies, but can be up to 2 hours

ADVANTAGES

• Family-centered as parents play an active role

• Based on a team approach, designed for use by a variety of disciplines, and applied in a variety of settings

• All data recording forms, parent and health record forms, and documentation forms included in the kit along with all test items, an administration manual, foundation/study guide, and additional readings

• Training kit available that includes a leader's guide and three videotapes

• IDA readings included in kit provide a sound base of knowledge to inexperienced practioners

LIMITATIONS

• Psychometric qualities are relatively weak

• Requires excessive preparation

• Few items in each domain; thus, a child may be heavily penalized for not showing a particular skill

(continued)

(*continued*)
• Ambiguous passing criteria for some items
• Wide range of ages used to determine percent delay

ORDERING INFORMATION

Riverside Publishing Company
8420 Bryn Mawr Avenue
Chicago, IL 60631

INFANT DEVELOPMENTAL SCREENING SCALE (IDSS)

W. Jane Proctor

PURPOSE

To determine developmental status of newborns

AGE RANGE

Normal and at-risk infants between 38 and 42 weeks gestational age; can also be used
sequentially on infants from 32 to 40 weeks gestational age

AREAS TESTED

Behavioral
Posture/movements
Reflexes

PSYCHOMETRIC CHARACTERISTICS

Criterion-referenced
Interrater reliability: percent agreement = 0.83 (habituation) to 0.96 (abnormal
posture/movements, reflexes)
Predictive valididty: proportion of children with at-risk or delayed scores on BSID
demonstrated significant linear trend with IDSS score
Sensitivity: 0.94
Specificity: 0.32

ADMINISTRATION

Summary scores are obtained for each area. Cut-off scores for each area categorize children
as normal, questionable, or high risk. Reflexes are scored as present/weak,
present/normal, or exaggerated. Reflex summary score is noted as 1 (optimal) to 5
(abnormal) depending on the number of exaggerated responses, clonus, and
asymmetries.

TIME REQUIRED

15–20 minutes

ADVANTAGES

• Simple administration and scoring procedures
• Behavioral items take into consideration cardiorespiratory responses and posture

LIMITATIONS

• Criteria are broad based
• 12 reflexes, including Moro, may be invasive and unnecesary
• Lacks adequate psychometric data
• Lacks published research regarding test development or theoretical support

(*continued*)

(continued)
ORDERING INFORMATION
Therapy Skill Builders
19500 Bulverde Road
San Antonio, TX 78259

INFANT NEUROBIOLOGICAL INTERNATIONAL BATTERY (INFANIB)

Patricia H. Ellison

PURPOSE

To distinguish infants with normal neuromotor function from those with abnormal findings and to predict need for follow-up treatment

AGE RANGE

1- to 18-month-old at-risk infants and toddlers, especially those born prematurely

AREAS TESTED

Spasticity

Vestibular function

Head and trunk control

French angles

Legs

PSYCHOMETRIC CHARACTERISTICS

Criterion-referenced

Internal consistency: Alpha for total score = 0.88 for infants <8 months, 0.43 for infants >8 months; 0.91 for total group

Interrater reliability: Pearson r = 0.97 for total test score

Test-retest reliability: Pearson r = 0.95

Predictive validity: spasticity and head and trunk subscales at 6 months highly predictive of cerebral palsy at 12 months (86.8% and 87.1%, respectively)

ADMINISTRATION

Individually administered with procedures for administering items described in text, but scoring procedures are on score sheet. Scores are calculated using corrected ages. Ages are grouped into four age "bins." Observed performance of infant compared with criteria in the four age groups. Scoring is based on how different the performance of the infant is compared with the expected performance at corrected age. Scores summed for each subscale and total test. Total scores are compared with cut-off points in three age groups and interpreted as abnormal, transient, or normal.

TIME REQUIRED

20–30 minutes

ADVANTAGES

- Manual contains excellent photographs, descriptions, and examples of infants (normal and abnormal) performing each item
- One-page scoring system

(continued)

(continued)

LIMITATIONS

- It is unclear how cut-off points were derived and why they are based on age groupings that are different from item age groupings
- Scoring procedures have some degree of subjectivity
- Manual contains superfluous information on reporting findings

ORDERING INFORMATION

Therapy Skill Builders
19500 Bulverde Road
San Antonio, TX 78259

INSIDE THE HAWAII EARLY LEARNING PROFILE (INSIDE-HELP)
Stephanie Parks

PURPOSE

To provide definitions and guidelines for administration and scoring of skills and to serve as a reference for all the HELP curriculum and assessment materials

AGE RANGE

Birth–36 months

AREAS TESTED

Regulatory/sensory organization

Cognition

Language

Gross motor

Fine motor

Social-emotional

Self-help

PSYCHOMETRIC CHARACTERISTICS

Criterion-referenced

Reviewed by early intervention programs in 35 states and 7 countries

Field tested on 200 infants to determine hierarchical ranking of items

ADMINISTRATION

Items can be observed in either a structured format or free play, with either the parent or professional interacting with the child. Items are scored as present, not present, or emerging. Additionally, it can be noted if the item was completed in an atypical way. The items within each strand are hierarchically oriented following a neuromaturational sequence. An approximate age range can be determined by the age level in the developmental strand at which the child completes all but two skills.

TIME REQUIRED

45–90 minutes

ADVANTAGES

- Written with the intent to comply with federal guidelines for family-centered assessment
- Allows credit for emerging skills

(continued)

(continued)
- The most widely used form of curriculum assessment
- The assessment is linked to HELP intervention strategies and cross-referenced to other HELP materials designed to aid in intervention
- Conceptual strands are advantageous for identifying strengths and needs for program planning
- Provides family-friendly interpretation of strand concepts, assessments, and purpose
- Computer software program available to track information and develop intervention strategies
- There is also HELP for preschoolers

LIMITATIONS
- Does not result in a standard score; therefore, must be used in conjunction with a standardized test if standardized scores are required for eligibility purposes
- Lacks research to establish validity and reliability
- Guidelines for estimating age equivalents are not provided, although the manual states that approximate developmental age levels can be determined

ORDERING INFORMATION
VORT Corporation
PO Box 60132
Palo Alto, CA 94306

MOVEMENT ASSESSMENT BATTERY FOR CHILDREN (MOVEMENT ABC)
Sheila E. Henderson and David A. Sugden

PURPOSE
To identify and describe impairments of motor function in children

AGE RANGE
4–12 years

AREAS TESTED
Performance Test
- Manual dexterity
- Ball skills
- Static and dynamic balance

Movement ABC Checklist
- Items that are part of daily routine (activities of daily living [ADL], mobility within environment, game playing)
- Takes into consideration context of performance and spatial and temporal dimensions
- Behavioral attributes

PSYCHOMETRIC CHARACTERISTICS
- Norm-referenced, standardized on 400 children in the United States

Test-retest reliability: Performance Test: percent agreement of items: 0.62 for item four at age band two to 1.0 for item seven at age band one; Checklist: r = 0.89 for total score, 0.88 for section one, 0.84 for section two, 0.77 for section three, and 0.76 for section four

(continued)

(continued)

Concurrent validity: r = −0.53 between Performance Test and BOTMP

Discriminative validity: significant difference in scores obtained in Performance Test between children with learning disabilities and those without and between children born with low birthweights and those of appropriate birth weights

ADMINISTRATION

Checklist is completed by parents, teachers, or other professionals as part of daily routine and can be filled in over 1–2 weeks. The Performance Test is individually administered using standardized procedures and materials. The age band that is the same as the child's chronologic age is administered. Scoring scheme varies with task. Raw scores are converted to scaled scores for each category (manual dexterity, ball skills, static and dynamic balance). The total scaled score converts to the total impairment score (TIS). The TIS converts to the percentile norm.

TIME REQUIRED

20–40 minutes

ADVANTAGES

- Takes into consideration qualitative and quantitative data
- Items are interesting to the child
- Behavioral factors that may influence performance are recorded
- All materials are included in the kit except stopwatch and clipboard
- Intervention guidelines provided
- Checklist provides information on how well the child performs in a group
- Photographs of item administration help clarify instructions
- Guidelines provided to adapt tasks for intervention planning
- Can purchase checklist separate from test kit

LIMITATIONS

- Scoring varies from task to task
- Scaled score converts to a percentile rank only
- Limited number of items
- Expensive
- Validity studies are limited
- Scoring does not allow for incremental changes in function
- Cannot buy replacement pieces or manual separate from kit

ORDERING INFORMATION

The Psychological Corporation
19500 Bulverde Road
San Antonio, TX 78259

MOVEMENT ASSESSMENT OF INFANTS (MAI)

Lynnette S. Chandler, Mary S. Andrews, and Marcia W. Swanson

PURPOSE

To identify motor dysfunction in infants, especially those considered at-risk, and monitor the effects of physical therapy on infants whose motor behaviors are at or below 1 year of age

(continued)

(*continued*)

AGE RANGE

Birth–12 months

AREAS TESTED

Muscle tone

Reflexes

Automatic reactions

Volitional movement

PSYCHOMETRIC CHARACTERISTICS

Normative data available for 4- and 8-month-old infants

Criterion-referenced

Interrater reliability: Pearson r = 0.72, ICC = 0.91 for total risk

Test-retest reliability: Pearson = 0.76, ICC = 0.79

Discriminates between infants born at <32 weeks gestation from those born between 32 and 36 weeks gestation at 4 months corrected age

Predictive validity: correlation between MAI total risk score and BSID at 1 year of age: −0.32 to −0.42. MAI at 4 months correctly identified 73.5% of children with cerebral palsy at 3–8 years of age and 62.7% of those that did not have cerebral palsy. Seventeen items shown to be significant predictors of cerebral palsy (primarily from volitional movement subtest)

Specificity: 0.78 at 4 months, 0.64 at 8 months

Sensitivity: 0.83 at 4 months, 0.96 at 8 months

ADMINISTRATION

Each of the four areas has a rating scale. Items are scored numerically according to specific criteria described in the manual. Asymmetries and muscle tone distribution variations, if substantial, are included when determining the final score. A total risk score is calculated by summing the points earned on the four scales.

TIME REQUIRED

45–90 minutes for administration and scoring

ADVANTAGES

- Specifically designed to be used with high-risk infants
- Quantifies aspects of movement quality
- Large literature base on its use with at-risk populations

LIMITATIONS

- High-risk profiles for 4- and 8-month-old infants only
- Lengthy to administer
- Reliability is generally fair to good
- High rates of false-positive results have been documented
- Requires extensive handling of the child

ORDERING INFORMATION

Infant Movement Research
PO Box 4631
Rolling Bay, WA 98061

THE MILANI-COMPARETTI MOTOR DEVELOPMENT SCREENING TEST, 3RD EDITION (MC)

Milani-Comparetti and E.A. Gidoni (Wayne Stuberg, for revised edition)

PURPOSE
To identify motor dysfunction in infants

AGE RANGE
Birth–2 years

AREAS TESTED
Spontaneous motor behaviors: locomotion, sitting, standing

Evoked responses: equilibrium reactions, protective extension reactions, righting reactions, primitive reflexes

PSYCHOMETRIC CHARACTERISTICS
Norm-referenced, standardized on 312 children between 1 and 16 months of age living in Omaha, Nebraska

Interrater reliability: mean percent agreement: 0.89–0.95

Item interrater reliability: 0.79 (standing)–0.98 (hand grasp, body lying supine)

Test-retest reliability: mean percent agreement = 0.82–1.0

Item Test Retest Reliability: .80 (body lying supine)—1.0 (Moro, backward protective reaction, pull to sit, standing up from supine, locomotion), Kappa − 0.65 (Landau)–1.0

Specificity: 0.78–0.89

Sensitivity: 0.44–0.67

ADMINISTRATION
Individually administered; drawings and a description of performance expected at different age levels are provided for each item. The examiner manipulates the child and scores the item on a timeline. A total score is not obtained. Scoring method provides a comparison of the child's age with the item age level to determine delays.

TIME REQUIRED
10–15 minutes

ADVANTAGES
• No specialized equipment is required, except a cushion or tilt board to assess equilibrium reactions

• Figures of responses depicted on response sheet

• Helpful for describing a child's motor development

• A videotape demonstrating procedures is available

LIMITATIONS
• No formal method of presenting or interpreting results

• Test's ability to discriminate changes in motor development is decreased after 12 months of age

• Limited documentation on reliability levels using populations of children with various degrees of disabilities

(continued)

(continued)

• Not a predictor of motor outcome

• Test based on construct that the integration of primitive reflexes is necessary for expression of automatic reactions and that development of automatic reactions is necessary for antigravity control of posture and movement

• Test emphasizes the handling of the child to gain information on select behaviors

ORDERING INFORMATION

Media Resource Center
Meyer Children's Rehabilitation Institute
University of Nebraska Medical Center
444 South 44th Street
Omaha, NE 68131-3795

MILLER ASSESSMENT OF PRESCHOOLERS (MAP)
Lucy Jane Miller

PURPOSE

To identify children at risk for mild or moderate preacademic problems

AGE RANGE

2 years, 9 months–5 years, 8 months

AREAS TESTED

Sensory and motor: foundation, coordination

Cognitive: nonverbal and verbal

Combined: complex tasks

PSYCHOMETRIC CHARACTERISTICS

Norm-referenced

Interrater reliability: Pearson $r = 0.97$–0.99 on individual indices (except coordination index $= 0.84$); 0.98 for whole test

Test-retest reliability at 2-week interval: percent agreement: 81% for total test, 94% for nonverbal to 72% for coordination

Internal consistency: for whole test Spearman Brown $= 0.79$ and Guttman $= 0.79$

Content validity: correlation analysis of each item and index revealed that test items contributed significantly to the total test (<0.1 level); contribution of each index was fairly equal (0.64–0.77)

Concurrent: with Weschler Preschool and Primary Scale Intelligence $r = 0.27$; with Illinois Test of Prelinguistic Abilities $r = 0.31$

Construct: MAP identified 75% of children who had been previously identified as functionally delayed (excluding cerebral palsy, mental retardation, and autism) as at risk or suspect.

ADMINISTRATION

Individually administered using items provided in the kit. Child must perform all activities; parental report is not acceptable. Six specific criteria sheets are provided in the manual according to the child's age. Raw scores are converted to percentile scores relative to the child's age. Strengths and weaknesses can be determined in the five index areas.

(continued)

(*continued*)

TIME REQUIRED

20–30 minutes

ADVANTAGES

- Test items are novel and presented in a game-like fashion, making them fun for children
- All equipment is included in the test kit
- Cue sheets ease administration
- Easy and quick to administer
- Most items are the same in all age categories, but some items are age-specific
- Conservative scoring cut off to prevent false-positive results and mislabeling of children
- Color-coded scoring for ease in interpretation

LIMITATIONS

- Rather lengthy for a screening tool
- Does not provide a standard score
- Coordination necessary by examiner to maintain correct cue sheet and item score sheet as well as to administer test items
- Few recommendations made regarding training needed to increase reliability of examiners
- Training strongly encouraged for administration and interpretation of the extended version
- Questionable predictive validity and screening accuracy

ORDERING INFORMATION

The Foundation for Knowledge in Development
1855 West Union Avenue
Suite B-8
Englewood, CO 80110

NEONATAL BEHAVIORAL ASSESSMENT SCALE (NBAS)

T. Berry Brazelton and J. Kevin Nugent

PURPOSE

To describe an infant's interactions and behaviors within the context of a dynamic relationship with a caregiver

AGE RANGE

Full-term neonates 37–48 weeks postconceptual age; supplemental items are provided to test infants born before 37 weeks

AREAS TESTED

Habituation

Motor-oral

Truncal

Vestibular

Social-interactive

There are also nine supplemental items that can be used with infants born prematurely

(*continued*)

(*continued*)

PSYCHOMETRIC CHARACTERISTICS

Criterion-referenced

Interrater relibility: with training percent agreement of .90

Test-retest reliability: modest as day-to-day stability in a newborn is expected to be low

Validity: has been shown to discriminate among groups of infants based on a variety of factors such as culture, socioeconomic status, interuterine drug exposure, birthweight, gestational age, and neonatal complications

ADMINISTRATION

Individually administered between feedings in a darkened room. Infant must be in required state for each test item. Specific criteria provided on testing procedures and item administration sequence. Test items are administered with increasingly complex sensory inputs to monitor infant responses. Infant is given credit for most optimal response rather than typical response. Seven total cluster scores are obtained.

TIME REQUIRED

30–35 minutes to administer, 10–15 minutes to score

ADVANTAGES

- Provides wealth of information on individual differences and interaction patterns
- An additional set of scores for some items representing average performance has been devised
- Information on how practitioners have used the NBAS as a therapeutic intervention and in research
- Clusters helpful in identifying strengths and needs
- Training tape available

LIMITATIONS

- Infant's state of consciousness and examiner's abilities are pivotal to the examination
- Premature infants often do not tolerate entire examination
- A costly and lengthy training program recommended to become reliable in administration

ORDERING INFORMATION

Clinics in Developmental Medicine, No. 137
Cambridge University Press
40 W. 20th Street
New York, NY 10011

NEONATAL NEUROBEHAVIORAL EXAMINATION (NNE)

Andrew Morgan, Vera Koch, Vicki Lee, and Jean Aldag

PURPOSE

To determine neurobehavioral status of infants

AGE RANGE

32–42 weeks postconceptional age

AREAS TESTED

Tone and motor patterns
Primitive reflexes
Behavioral responses

(*continued*)

(continued)

PSYCHOMETRIC CHARACTERISTICS

Criterion-referenced tool standardized on a sample of 54 infants born full-term and 298 infants at high risk

Interrater reliability for full term infants: percent agreement = 0.88 for item agreement and 0.95 for section agreement

Predictive validity between NNE and PDMS: r = 0.003–0.169

Performance on test discriminates infants born full-term from those born preterm

ADMINISTRATION

The NNE score sheet contains line drawings and simple instructions. There is a three-point scoring system for each item. Item scores are summed to obtain section scores which are summed to obtain total score.

TIME REQUIRED

5–20 minutes

ADVANTAGES

- Quick to administer
- Line drawings aid administration
- Takes into consideration gestational age

LIMITATIONS

- Lacks standardized testing procedures
- Information available about the tool lacks details and is limitted in scope
- Little recent information in uses for the tool

ORDERING INFORMATION

Morgan, A. M., Koch, V., Lee, V., & Aldag, J. *Physical Therapy, 68,* 1352–1358.

NEONATAL ORAL MOTOR ASSESSMENT SCALE (NOMAS)

Murray A. Braun and Marjorie M. Palmer

PURPOSE

To screen for oral motor dysfunction in the neonate, distinguish infants with normal sucking from those with disorganization, identify infants with poor feeding abilities, and distinguish inefficient from efficient feeders

AGE RANGE

Neonate–3 months

AREAS TESTED

Rate

Rhythmicity

Consistency of degree of jaw excursion

Direction, range of motion, timing of tongue movement

Tongue configuration

(continued)

(continued)

PSYCHOMETRIC CHARACTERISTICS

Criterion-referenced

Interrater reliability: percent agreement = 0.63 (inconsistent degree of jaw depression) to 1.0 (asymmetry, lateral jaw deviation, jaw movements) and 0.63 (movements occur at rate of 1/sec) to 1.0 (asymmetry of tongue movements)

Test-retest reliability: Pearson r = 0.67–0.83; differentiates inefficient from efficient feeders in both nutritive and nonnutritive conditions

ADMINISTRATION

Observation of the infant during nonnutritive and then nutritive sucking. The items are divided into normal, disorganized, or dysfunctional categories. Each category is totaled. It is unclear what the total scores indicate on the most recently revised version. On the pilot version a score of 48 was considered normal, 43–47 some oral-motor disorganization, and 42 oral-motor dysfunction.

TIME REQUIRED

15 minutes

ADVANTAGES

- Differentiates among normal, disorganized, and dysfunctional infants
- Observation only
- No specialized equipment required except pacifier and bottle with the same nipple
- Provides structured observational format
- May be helpful in treatment planning

LIMITATIONS

- Operational definitions of scoring criterion limited
- Limited psychometric information
- Interpretation of scores very unclear
- Some definitions of jaw, tongue characteristics unclear

ORDERING INFORMATION

Palmer, M. M. (1993). Identification and management of the transitional suck pattern in premature infants. *Journal of Perinatal Neonatal Nursing, 7* (1), 66–75.

NEUROLOGICAL ASSESSMENT OF THE PRETERM AND FULLTERM BORN INFANT (NAPFI)

Lilly Dubowitz and Victor Dubowitz

PURPOSE

To document neurologic maturation or change in infants and to detect deviations in neurologic signs

AGE RANGE

Full-term infants up to the third day of life and preterm infants who are medically stable and can tolerate handling up to term gestation age

AREAS TESTED

Habituation

Movement and tone

(continued)

(*continued*)

Reflexes

Neurobehavioral

PSYCHOMETRIC CHARACTERISTICS

Criterion-referenced

Reliability has not been determined

Sensitivity: 0.65

Specificity: 0.91

ADMINISTRATION

Administer two-thirds of the way between feedings. Scoring yields a descriptive profile of the infant's responses to reflect different aspects of neurologic function. A cumulative score is not obtained. Infants are categorized as normal, abnormal, or borderline depending on tone, head control, or number of deviant signs seen on examination. The infant state is recorded for each item. Asymmetries are also recorded for the appropriate items.

TIME REQUIRED

10–15 minutes to perform examination and record findings

ADVANTAGES

• Quick and simple to administer

• Recording sheets contain instructions and illustrations of possible responses

• Applicable to both preterm and sick full-term infants

LIMITATIONS

• Limited psychometric data available, especially lack of reliability

• Although commonly used, there is limited literature on its applicability and psychometric properties

ORDERING INFORMATION

Clinics in Developmental Medicine, No. 79
Cambridge University Press
40 W. 20th Street
New York, NY 10011

NEUROLOGICAL EXAM OF THE FULL TERM INFANT
Heinz Prechtl

PURPOSE

To diagnose infants with neurologic abnormality and predict future neurologic problems. A screening test is also available that can be used to determine the need for further testing in low-risk infants

AGE RANGE

Full-term and preterm infants 38–42 weeks gestation

AREAS TESTED

Posture

Eyes

(*continued*)

(*continued*)

Power and passive movements

Spontaneous and voluntary movements

State

PSYCHOMETRIC CHARACTERISTICS

Norm-referenced

Interrater reliability (of states): percent agreement = 1.0; interrater: Pearson r = 0.70 (muscle tone) to 1.0 (state)

Discriminant validity (of states): age-related state changes

Predictive validity of syndrome classification to status at 1 year of age: 73%

Sensitivity: >80%

ADMINISTRATION

The test is divided into two parts: the observation period and the examination period. Items are presented in groups (prone, supine, prone suspension, vertical suspension) and scored as present or absent. Presence of an item is scored on a continuum based on intensity. The intensity criteria vary depending on the item. Asymmetries are also noted. Each item is state-based with optimum state noted for each item. No total score is obtained, but neurologic findings frequently appear in particular combinations identified as four syndromes: apathy syndrome, hyperexcitability syndrome, hemisyndrome, and comatose syndrome.

TIME REQUIRED

30–60 minutes

ADVANTAGES

• Well-standardized instructions for administration

• Asymmetric responses and reflexes noted

• Emphasis on state control

• Manual provides information on the significance of each item

• Screening tool is also available

LIMITATIONS

• Long and complex to score

• Abbreviated test decreases validity

• Predictive validity of single examination is low

• Emphasis on reflexes

ORDERING INFORMATION

Clinics in Developmental Medicine, No. 63
Cambridge University Press
40 W. 20th Street
New York, NY 10011

NEONATAL INDIVIDUALIZED DEVELOPMENTAL CARE AND ASSESSMENT PROGRAM (NIDCAP)

Heidelise Als

PURPOSE

To document an infant's physiological and behavioral responses to the environment and caregiving procedures

(*continued*)

(continued)

AGE RANGE

Neonates–4 weeks postterm

AREAS TESTED

Autonomic

Motor

Attention

PSYCHOMETRIC CHARACTERISTICS

Criterion-referenced

Interrater reliability: percent agreement >0.85 for trained administrators

ADMINISTRATION

Systematic observation of the preterm or full-term infant in the nursery or home during caregiving routines or manipulations performed by caregiver. Caregiving suggestions and environmental adaptations are based on observations.

TIME REQUIRED

60 minutes (20 minutes before caregiving, 20 minutes during caregiving, and 20 minutes after caregiving)

ADVANTAGES

• Can be used in a variety of settings and by a variety of personnel
• Observation only
• Provides wealth of information on the infant's reaction to internal and external stimuli
• Observations can be linked directly to intervention suggestions
• Excellent teaching tool regarding behaviors of infants

LIMITATIONS

• Lengthy to administer
• Majority of items on observation sheet are subjective
• Depending on the infant, may not observe the variety of behaviors infant uses; thus, may require multiple observations to develop comprehensive plans

ORDERING INFORMATION

National NIDCAP Training Center
Enders Pediatric Research Laboratories
The Children's Hospital
320 Longwood Avenue
Boston, MA 02115

ORAL MOTOR/FEEDING RATING SCALE

Judy Michaels Jelm

PURPOSE

To document oral motor/feeding patterns and feeding function

AGE RANGE

1 year–adulthood

AREAS TESTED

Oral motor/feeding patterns: lip/cheek movement, tongue movement, jaw movement

(continued)

(continued)

Related areas of feeding function: self-feeding, adaptive feeding equipment, diet adaptation, position, sensitivity, food retention, swallowing, oral-facial structures

ADMINISTRATION

Observation of the individual during the feeding of a typical meal. The lip/cheek, tongue, and jaw movements are noted on a six-point descriptive scale during eight feeding behaviors appropriate for the age of the individual: breast, bottle, spoon, cup, biting soft food, biting hard food, chewing, and straw drinking. Two optional areas are available to note influence on respiration/phonation patterns and gross/fine motor skill development.

TIME REQUIRED

Varies depending on age and severity of disability

Can be administered in whole or in part and over a course of meals

A typical meal takes between 20 and 40 minutes to complete

ADVANTAGES

• Organizes observations of oral motor behaviors

LIMITATIONS

• No information on how this scale assists in differentiating children with various oral-motor patterns or how it is related to intervention
• Lacks psychometric characteristics
• Lacks research

ORDERING INFORMATION

Therapy Skill Builders
19500 Bulverde Road
San Antonio, TX 78259

PEABODY DEVELOPMENT MOTOR SCALES (PDMS)

M. Rhonda Folio and Rebecca R. Fewell

PURPOSE

To determine the level of motor skill acquisition, detect small changes in motor development in children with known motor delays or disabilities, and assist in programming for children with disabilities

AGE RANGE

1–72 months

AREAS TESTED

Gross Motor Scale

• Reflexes
• Stationary
• Locomotion
• Object manipulation

Fine Motor Scale

• Grasping
• Visual-motor integration

(continued)

(continued)

PSYCHOMETRIC CHARACTERISTICS

Norm-referenced, standardized on 2003 children stratified by Census Bureau data

Standard error of measurement (rounded values): gross motor and fine motor scales: 1 for all age levels except for two 2's in 36–47 months; composite scales: range between 2 (ages 0–11, 48–59, and 60–72 months) and 5 (ages 36–47 months)

Test-retest reliability: Pearson r = 0.82–0.94 gross motor scale; 0.87–0.92 fine motor scale

Interrater reliability: Pearson r = 0.97–0.99 gross motor scale; 0.98 fine motor scale

Construct validity: gross motor and fine motor: 0.79; stationary, locomotion, reflexes, and object manipulation subtests to gross motor construct: 0.78, 0.85, 0.63, and 0.63, respectively; visual-motor integration and grasping subtests to fine motor construct: 0.83 and 0.65, respectively

Content: Pearson r = 0.35–0.69

Concurrent: Pearson r = 0.84 gross motor scale with PDMS, 0.91 fine motor with PDMS

ADMINISTRATION

Individually administered test using standardized procedures. Some test items are included in the kit, most are not. Items are scored on a three-point scale. Raw scores convert to age equivalent (AE), percentiles, and standard scores. Standard scores convert to three global indexes (composites) of motor performance: gross motor (GM), fine motor (FM), and total motor quotients. Each skill that a child has mastered is plotted on a chart that indicates the age at which 50% of the normalization population passed the item.

TIME REQUIRED

45–60 minutes

ADVANTAGES

- General guidelines provided for modifying test procedures for children with disabilities
- Distinguishes between gross and fine motor skills
- Test broken down into different areas to identify strengths and needs
- Scaled scoring system available to measure progress in children with known disabilities or delays
- Scoring system takes into consideration emerging skills
- Interpretation of subtest standard scores chart
- Discrepancy analysis procedure to determine if differences seen in subtests are significantly different
- Scoring booklet has abbreviated directions and scoring criteria for each item

LIMITATIONS

- Test does not include quality of movement
- Examiner required to provide majority of test materials
- Some test materials are not easily acquired and descriptions not precisely specified
- Motor activities program book may encourage teaching test items

ORDERING INFORMATION

Riverside Publishing Company
8420 Bryn Mawr Avenue
Chicago, IL 60631

CHAPTER 3

PEDIATRIC EVALUATION OF DISABILITY INVENTORY (PEDI)
Stephen M. Haley, Wendy J. Coster, Larry H. Ludlow, Jane T. Haltiwarger, and Peter J. Andrellas

PURPOSE
To determine functional capabilities and performance, monitor progress in functional skill performance, and evaluate therapeutic or rehabilitative program outcome in children with disabilities

AGE RANGE
6 months–7 years, 6 months

AREAS TESTED
Self care: eating, grooming, dressing, bathing, toileting

Mobility: transfers, indoors and outdoors mobility

Social function: communication, social interaction, household and community tasks

Modification scale and caregiver assistance scale

PSYCHOMETRIC CHARACTERISTICS
Norm-referenced, standardized on 412 typically developing children and their families and 3 small samples of children with disabilities

Internal consistency: Cronbach's Alpha = 0.95 (caregiver assistance scale, social function)–0.99 (functional skills scale, self-care)

Interrater reliability: ICC = 0.96–0.99 for nonclinical sample on caregiver assistance scale and 0.79–1.00 on modification scale, ICC = 0.84–1.00 for clinical sample

Concurrent validity: r = 0.73 between functional skills scale and BDIST for total sample, 0.70 for children with disabilities, and 0.81 for nondisabled; r = 0.71 between caregiver assistance scale and BDIST for total sample, 0.73 for children with disabilities and 0.62 for nondisabled; r = 0.92 between total functional skills scale and total WeeFim and 0.93 between total caregiver assistance and total WeeFim

Discriminant validity: 59% for caregiver assistance scale for self-care at 2–5 years of age to 100% for the functional skills scale, mobility domain in children older than age 5 in the typically developing children group; 47% for functional skills scale, social function domain to 75% for functional skills scale, self-care domain in the clinical sample

ADMINISTRATION
Administered by parent report, structured interview, or through professional observation of a child's functional behavior. The functional skills scale has a binary scoring system, and the caregiver assistance scale is a six-point continuum scale (independent to total assistance). The modification scale is a frequency count of type of adaptations used. Standard scores and scaled scores can be obtained for the functional skills scale and the caregiver assistance scale.

TIME REQUIRED
20–60 minutes to administer and score depending on the child's age, level of function, and method of administration

ADVANTAGES
- Reliable and valid assessment of functional performance in children with cognitive and physical disabilities
- Focus on function and level of independence

(continued)

(continued)

- Children with disabilities receive credit for mastery of certain components of complex functional skills
- Flexibility: each PEDI scale is self-contained and can be used separately or in combination depending on the child's needs
- Computer software program available to aid in scoring
- Measures amount of caregiver assistance required to accomplish tasks

LIMITATIONS

- Therapist and caregiver perceptions of the child can differ on selected PEDI items
- Requires additional reliability and validity studies on larger samples with more diverse disabilities

ORDERING INFORMATION

Center for Rehabilitation Effectiveness
Boston University
Sargent College of Health and Rehabilitation Sciences
635 Commonwealth avenue
Boston, MA 02215

SCALES OF INDEPENDENT BEHAVIOR—REVISED (SIB-R)
Robert H. Bruininks, Richard W. Woodcock, Richard F. Weatherman, and Bradley K. Hill

PURPOSE

To measure functional independence and adaptive functioning in school, home, employment, and community settings

AGE RANGE

3 months–90+ years

AREAS TESTED

Motor skills
Social interaction and communication skills
Personal living skills
Community living skills
Problem Behavior Scale
- Internalized maladaptive behavior
- Asocial maladaptive behavior
- Externalized maladaptive behavior

PSYCHOMETRIC CHARACTERISTICS

Norm-referenced, standardized on 2182 typically developing people from 3 months to 90 years of age

Test-retest reliability: $r = 0.69$ (asocial maladaptive index at 10–11 years)–0.98 (full scale)

Internal consistency: $r = 0.70$ (home/community orientation)–0.99 (full scale)

Internal consistency for children with mental retardation: $r = 0.92$ (money and value)–0.99 (full scale)

(continued)

CHAPTER 3

(continued)

Interrater reliability: r = 0.58 (toileting)–0.95 (full scale)

Interrater reliability for children with mental retardation: r = 0.57 (internalized maladaptive)–0.97 (motor skills)

Scores differentiated individuals with learning disabilities, mental retardation, and behavior disorders from typically developing individuals

ADMINISTRATION

Individually administered via interview with or checklist completed by respondent familiar with the person being assessed. Raw scores for the short form, early development form, and adaptive behavior full scale convert to W scores (special transformation of Rasch ability scale), age-equivalent scores, cluster scores, relative mastery indexes, adaptive behavior skill levels, percentile ranks, and standard scores. Raw scores for the problem behavior scale convert to support scores that combine adaptive behavior and problem behavior to determine overall intensity of resources, needed support, and supervision.

TIME REQUIRED

Adaptive behavior full scale: 45–60 minutes

Short form scale: 15–20 minutes

Early development scale: 15–20 minutes

Problem behavior scale: 10 minutes

ADVANTAGES

- Provides information on person's current level of functioning at home and in the community
- Objective assessment supplemented by open-ended questions that provide information that can be used to determine goals and program objectives unique to each individual
- Statistically and conceptually linked to the Woodcock-Johnson Psycho-Education Battery; thus, can be used to compare individual's functional independence, problem behaviors, cognitive ability, achievement, and interests
- Very flexible administration
- Age-equivalent scoring tables placed directly in the response booklets
- Screening forms include one specifically for children younger than the developmental age of 8 years
- Administration and scoring of the SIB do not require extensive training
- Nationally standardized for infants, children, and adults
- Optional computer program available for scoring and interpreting the SIB-R
- Is a component of the Adaptive Living Skills Assessment Intervention System, which links assessment to curriculum objectives

LIMITATIONS

- Item scoring and score conversion are tedious, thus increasing the opportunity for scoring errors
- Adaptive behavior full scale is lengthy to administer
- No predictive validity studies available

ORDERING INFORMATION

Riverside Publishing Co.
8420 Bryn Mawr Avenue
Chicago, IL 60603

SCHOOL FUNCTION ASSESSMENT (SFA)

Wendy Coster, Theresa Deeney, Jane Haltiwanger, and Stephen Haley

PURPOSE

To assess function and guide program planning for students with disabilities within the educational environment

AGE RANGE

Children with disabilities attending grades K–6

AREAS TESTED

Participation: classroom, playground/recess, transportation, bathroom/toileting, transitions to and from class, meal/snack times

Task supports: types of assistance from adults; adaptations or modifications to the environment on each of the scales in the activity performance part yielding four scales (physical task assistance, physical task adaptations, cognitive/behavioral task assistance, and cognitive/behavioral task adaptations)

Activity performance: student's performance of specific school-related functional activities

Physical tasks: travel, maintaining and changing positions, recreational movement, manipulation with movement, using materials, setup and cleanup, eating and drinking, hygiene, clothing management, up/down stairs, written work, and computer and equipment use

Cognitive/behavioral tasks: functional communication, memory/understanding, following social conventions, compliance with adult directives and school rules, task behavior/completion, positive interaction, behavior regulation, safety, and personal care awareness

PSYCHOMETRIC CHARACTERISTICS

Criterion-referenced, standardized on 678 children representing those receiving regular education and those receiving special education

Internal consistency: Cronbach's Alpha: 0.92–0.98

Test-retest reliability: Pearson $r = 0.80$–0.98; ICC $= 0.80$–0.98

Construct validity: (a) different activity settings reflect different degrees of difficulty; (b) multiple regression analysis indicates that there are setting-specific key tasks

ADMINISTRATION

Judgment-based, format gathering information from a variety of individuals involved in the student's education. Each item of each part must be rated to obtain a raw score. Ratings must reflect typical performance and be assigned by comparing the student to his or her same age/grade peers. Each item is rated based on adequacy of performance, not method used unless otherwise stated. Whenever the assistance scale is completed in part II, the corresponding adaptation scale should also be completed. Raw scores convert to criterion scores, which can be compared to cut-off scores. Standard error of measurement is also obtained.

TIME REQUIRED

Varies based on familiarity with system, but may take up to 2 hours to complete

ADVANTAGES

- Content specifically relevant for children with physical or sensory impairments
- Requires input from a variety of respondents, thus yielding information about a student across domains and environments

(continued)

(continued)

- Judgment is based on *typical* performance rather than optimal
- Total and individual scale scores are obtained; thus, pattern of strengths and weaknesses can be determined
- Designed to be used in integrated settings
- Specific examples are given for each rating

LIMITATIONS

- Requires collaboration and coordination among team members to obtain valid information
- Does not determine the cause of limitations
- Can be time-consuming

ORDERING INFORMATION

Therapy Skill Builders
19500 Bulverde Road
San Antonio, TX 78259

SENSORY INTEGRATION INVENTORY FOR INDIVIDUALS WITH DEVELOPMENTAL DISABILITIES—REVISED (SII-R)

Judith E. Reisman and Bonnie Hanschu

PURPOSE

To identify sensory integrative dysfunction

AGE RANGE

Children and adults with developmental disabilities

AREAS TESTED

Tactile

Vestibular

Proprioceptive

General reactions

PSYCHOMETRIC CHARACTERISTICS

No psychometric characteristics reported in manual

ADMINISTRATION

Therapist-completed through direct knowledge or through semistructured interview with direct caregivers. Responses are indicative of typical behavior. No score is determined. Judgment of presence of sensory integrative dysfunction is based on pattern of responses and relies on interpretive skill of therapist administrator.

TIME REQUIRED

30 minutes

ADVANTAGES

- Provides structure system to collect clinical information and information on behaviors that may have a sensory integration base

(continued)

(continued)
- Can be used with adults with a known developmental disability
- Judgment is based on typical behavior of client

LIMITATIONS
- No research described to support purpose of test, selection of items, or basis of judgment
- Depends on the skill of the therapist to analyze information
- Items scored subjectively from subjective criteria

ORDERING INFORMATION
PDP Press
12015 North July Avenue
Hugo, MN 55038

SENSORY INTEGRATION AND PRAXIS TESTS (SIPT)
A. Jean Ayres

PURPOSE
To measure the sensory integration processes that underlie learning and behavior

AGE RANGE
4 years–8 years, 11 months

AREAS TESTED
Form and space perception
Somatic and vestibular sensory processing
Praxis
Bilateral integration and sequencing

PSYCHOMETRIC CHARACTERISTICS
Norm-referenced
Interrater reliability: Pearson $r = 0.94$–0.99 for all major tests
Test-retest reliability: at 1- to 2-week intervals: 4 of 17 subtests fall below 0.60 postrotary
   nystagmus, 2 of the somatosensory (kinesthesia, localization of tactile stimulation),
   1 visual test (figure-ground perception), all others >0.60
Concurrent validity: not applicable because there are no comparable SI and praxis tests
   covering the same age range

ADMINISTRATION
Each of 17 subtests has specific instructions. These include specific verbal instructions, rules for
   demonstration of tasks, and criteria for discontinuance. Scores for each section are recorded
   on the Western Pyschological Service (WPS) Test Report answer sheets and sent to the WPS,
   where results are computurized. Standard deviation and percentile scores are given

TIME REQUIRED
2 hours for the entire battery (2 testing sittings for entire battery are recommended)

ADVANTAGES
- Test has minimal dependence on linguistic competence: can use nonverbal communication
- Validity studies indicate use to differentiate diagnostic groups
- All scoring is completed by the WPS, and a detailed report explaining SIPT results is provided

(continued)

(continued)

LIMITATIONS
- Lengthy time to administer
- Extensive training to administer
- Special equipment necessary
- Not to be used with children with severe neuromotor dysfunction
- Expensive
- Few follow-up studies have been conducted to support reliability and validity
- Test-retest reliability weak for four of the subtests

ORDERING INFORMATION
Western Pyschological Services
12031 Wilshire Boulevard
Los Angeles, CA 90025

SENSORY PERFORMANCE ANALYSIS (SPA)
Eileen W. Richter and Patricia C. Montgomery

PURPOSE
To assess the quality of a child's performance for program planning and to document change over time

AGE RANGE
5–21 years

AREAS TESTED
Rolling
Belly crawling
Bat the ball from three-point
Kneeling balance
Pellets in a bottle
Paper and pencil task
Scissor task
16 sensorimotor (performance) components are analyzed for each task

PSYCHOMETRIC CHARACTERISTICS
Criterion-referenced
Test-retest reliability: Pearson $r = 0.89$–0.97
Interrater reliability: Pearson $r = 0.15$ (STNR)–0.91 (motor planning)

ADMINISTRATION
Each task is analyzed according to the sensorimotor performance components specific for each task. Low scores (<4) on a sensorimotor component indicates dysfunction, and treatment should be considered. Performance items are grouped according to sensorimotor components, and areas to be addressed in therapy are identified.

(continued)

(continued)

TIME REQUIRED

30–45 minutes

ADVANTAGES

- Attempts to quantify items/tasks that are often considered clinical observations
- Specifically designed for use with children and young adults with developmental disabilities
- Case studies with sample treatment plans and reports provided in text
- Required equipment is commonly found in therapy departments
- Scoring system easily understood
- Primarily used for intervention planning and follow-up
- Eight tasks of commonly identified areas of neurologic function make up a quick screen

LIMITATIONS

- Poor interrater reliability on three component subscales: ATNR, STNR, and tactile processing
- Criteria for item selection not clear and appear subjective
- Criteria for interpretation of scores are subjective, not well defined, and may lead to overreferral to intervention

ORDERING INFORMATION

PDP Press, PDP Products
12015 North July Avenue
Hugo, MN 55038

SENSORY PROFILE

Winnie Dunn

PURPOSE

To determine which sensory processes contribute to performance strengths and barriers in a child's daily life

AGE RANGE

5–10 years; there is information on using it for children 3–4 years

AREAS TESTED

Sensory processing: responses to basic sensory systems (auditory, visual, vestibular, touch, multisensory, oral)

Modulation (sensory processing related to endurance and tone, body position and movement, movement affecting activity level, sensory inputs affecting emotional responses, visual input affecting emotional responses and activity level)

Behavioral/emotional responses (emotional/social responses, behavioral outcomes, items indicating thresholds for response)

ADMINISTRATION

Parent-completed questionnaire.

TIME REQUIRED

30 minutes

(continued)

(continued)

ADVANTAGES

- Family-centered/family-friendly
- Links sensory processing to every day skills
- Provides a theoretical construct to determine areas of strength/weakness
- Screener available

LIMITATIONS

- School-age children only
- Conceptual model may be difficult to understand initially
- Need to reformat scores to determine areas of need and to classify based on areas grouped

ORDERING INFORMATION

The Psychological Corporation
19500 Bulverde Road
San Antonio, TX 78259

TEST OF GROSS MOTOR DEVELOPMENT—2 (TGMD2)
Dale Ulrich

PURPOSE

To determine a child's acquisition of aspects of selected gross motor tasks

AGE RANGE

3–10 years

AREAS TESTED

Locomotion

Object control

Each item contains three to four specific performance criteria indicative of maturity of skill

PSYCHOMETRIC CHARACTERISTICS

Norm- and criterion-referenced

Normative sample was 1208

Reliability: locomotor subtest average 0.85; object control subtest 0.88; gross motor composite 0.91

SEM is 1 at every age interval for both subtests and 4 or 5 for the composite score at each age interval

Coefficient alpha for selected subgroups are all above 0.90 for the subtest and the composite

Time sampling reliability coefficients range from 0.84 to 0.96

Validity: Content-description, criterion-prediction, and construct-identification validity indicate that the test identifies children who are significantly behind their peers in gross motor development

ADMINISTRATION

Individually administered test using tester-supplied materials described in the manual and standardized procedures. Each skill is delineated into four behavioral components (performance criteria). Each component is scored with a 1 if observed for two out of three

(continued)

(continued)

trials or a zero if not observed. A practice and three test trials are given for each item. Performance components are arranged from least to most mature within each skill. Raw scores convert to percentiles, standard scores, and developmental quotients based on age.

TIME REQUIRED

15–30 minutes

ADVANTAGES

- Provides information on component skill development of tasks typically performed by young children during play
- Provides information on the age most children complete all aspects of each skill
- Minimal amount of equipment is required
- Each skill and performance component operationally defined
- Diagrams of items
- Descriptive ratings of standard scores given for each subtest and total score

LIMITATIONS

- Little research reported on its use with children with various disabilities
- Some areas of gross motor skills not sufficiently addressed (i.e., balance)
- Best used for intervention purposes rather than diagnostic, eligibility, or placement decisions

ORDERING INFORMATION

PRO-ED
5341 Industrial Oaks Boulevard
Austin, TX 78735

TEST OF SENSORY FUNCTION IN INFANTS (TSFI)

Georgia DeGangi and Stanley Greenspan

PURPOSE

To determine sensory processing and reactivity in infants to assist in diagnosing sensory processing dysfunction

AGE RANGE

4–18 months

AREAS TESTED

Reactivity to tactile deep pressure
Adaptive motor function
Visual-tactile integration
Ocular motor control
Reactivity to vestibular stimulation

PSYCHOMETRIC CHARACTERISTICS

Criterion-referenced
Interrater reliability: ICC = 0.88 (adaptive motor)–0.99 (reactivity to vestibular stimulation)
Decision consistency: p_o = 81% (reactivity to tactile deep pressure)–96% (visual-tactile integration and ocular-motor control)

(continued)

(continued)

Test-retest reliability: Pearson r = 0.26 (reactivity to vestibular stimulation)–0.96 (ocular-motor control)

Decision: false normal rate for total test score 14–45%; false delayed rate for total test score 11–19%

Construct: intercorrelations range from a low of r = 0.02 for reactivity to tactile deep pressure and reactivity to vestibular stimulation to 0.47 for adaptive-motor and visual-tactile integration; each subtest to total test ranged from r = 0.30 (tactile deep pressure) to r = 0.74 (adaptive motor)

Criterion: to Bayley Scales of Infant Development, Motor Scale r 5 0.160, Mental Scale r = −0.204, Bates Infant Characteristics Questionnaire r = 0.015, Fagen test r = 0.006

ADMINISTRATION

Individually administered to infants sitting on caregiver's lap (except for vestibular subtest) with materials provided in the kit. Items are presented in a set format from least intrusive (tactile-deep pressure) to most intrusive (reactivity to vestibular stimulation). Within each subtest the items are again presented from least intrusive to most intrusive. If infant expresses stranger anxiety, caregiver may be coached in the item administration. According to the authors, for diagnostic decision-making the TSFI is most accurate for identifying infants without sensory processing disorders from 4–18 months of age and infants with sensory dysfunction from 10–18 months of age.

TIME REQUIRED

25 minutes to administer and score

ADVANTAGES

- First instrument designed to screen infants for sensory dysfunction
- May prove useful in predicting subtle sensory integration dysfunction during infancy
- Most items can be scored while the infant is held in a caregiver's lap
- All test items are included in the test kit
- Test form is clear and contains instructions

LIMITATIONS

- Some items can be intrusive; thus, the infant may not tolerate all items
- Stranger anxiety is a confounding factor
- More effective in detecting infants without sensory processing dysfunction that those with processing difficulties
- Norming population is relatively small and is not nationally representative
- Based on psychometric data, best suited to be used with infants older than 7 months of age

ORDERING INFORMATION

Western Psychological Services
12031 Wilshire Boulevard
Los Angeles, CA 90025

TEST OF VISUAL-MOTOR SKILLS—REVISED (TVMS-R)

Morrison F. Gardner

PURPOSE

To document visual motor functioning

(continued)

(continued)

AGE RANGE

3–13 years, 11 months

AREAS TESTED

Visual-motor skills

PSYCHOMETRIC CHARACTERISTICS

Norm referenced

Internal consistency: Cronbach's Alpha: total design −0.90 across age groups; Kuder-Richardson: individual characteristics for each age level: 0.77–0.86; across age levels 0.92; SEM: ranged from 5.61 to 7.19, with a median of 6.27 for standard scores

Construct validity: subscale intercorrelations: 0.29–0.68

Concurrent validity: Bender Gestalt: 0.33 (age 9), 0.61 (age 5), median 0.60; VMI: 0.33 (age 12) to 0.59 (age 7), median 0.51

ADMINISTRATION

Administered individually or in a group. The child is asked to copy all 23 designs with a pencil without erasing. If designs become too difficult for the child, the test can be terminated after four consecutive failures. A score for number of errors and number of accuracies is calculated and converted to a standard score, scaled score, percentile rank, and stanine score. An age-equivalent can be determined for accuracies. Standard scores are derived for the total test and the individual subscales (eight classifications).

TIME REQUIRED

Untimed but generally completed within 10 minutes.

ADVANTAGES

- Easy and quick to administer
- Inexpensive to purchase, administer, and score
- Can be administered to an individual or a group
- Items are in order of increasing complexity
- Has a companion guide, "Visual-Motor Development Remediation Activities"

LIMITATIONS

- Limited geographical distribution of standardization population
- Description of standardization population does not include gender and ethnicity
- Requires the use of a protractor to score
- Scoring may take longer than 30 minutes
- Moderate reliability and validity

ORDERING INFORMATION

Psychological and Educational Publications, Inc.
PO Box 520
Hydesville, CA 95547-0520

TEST OF VISUAL-PERCEPTUAL SKILLS (NON-MOTOR)— REVISED (TVPS-R)

Morrison F. Gardner

PURPOSE

To determine visual perceptual skills

(continued)

(continued)

AGE RANGE

4–12 years

AREAS TESTED

Visual discrimination

Visual memory

Visual spatial relationships

Visual form constancy

Visual sequential memory

Visual figure ground

Visual closure

PSYCHOMETRIC CHARCTERISTICS

Norm-referenced

Internal consistency: subtest reliabilities are split-half: alpha coefficients ranging from 0.27 to 0.80, median reliability coefficients across age levels 0.42 to 0.61, and total score 0.83 to 0.91

Diagnostic validity: children with learning disabilities scored well below the average

Concurrent validity: correlation coefficients 0.11–0.45 when correlating subtest standard scores from final form to standard scores of subtests of the Test of Academic Achievement Skills, WISC-Third Edition, WPPSI-Revised, WRAT-Third Edition, Visual- Motor Skills-Revised, Test of Auditory Perceptual Skills-Revised, and Test of Non-Verbal Intelligence-Second Edition

ADMINISTRATION

Child chooses a match for the stimulus form from a multiple choice array. The child points to response, receiving one point for each correct answer. There are discontinuation criteria for each subtest. Raw scores are converted to standard scores (perceptual quotients, percentile ranks, and median perceptual ages) for each subtest and the total test.

ADVANTAGES

• No special equipment needed to administer

• Easy to administer

• Yields specific information on seven areas of visual perception to determine the child's strengths and weaknesses

• Directions require only a minimum amount of language and can be given in any language or by gesture; answers may be given by pointing.

LIMITATIONS

• Sample distribution limited to one geographical area

• Poor predictive validity

• Lengthy to administer

• No test-retest reliability

ORDERING INFORMATION

Psychological and Educational Publications, Inc.

PO Box 520

Hydesville, CA 95547-0520

TODDLER & INFANT MOTOR EVALUATION (TIME)

Lucy Jane Miller and Gale H. Roid

PURPOSE

To identify those children with mild to severe motor problems, identify patterns of movement, evaluate motor development over time, plan intervention, and conduct treatment efficacy research

AGE RANGE

4 months–3.5 years

AREAS TESTED

Primary Subtests

- Mobility
- Motor organization
- Stability-functional performance
- Social-emotional abilities

Clinical Subtests

- Quality rating
- Component analysis
- Atypical positions

PSYCHOMETRIC CHARACTERISTICS

The primary subtests are norm-referenced

Internal consistency by age group: Cronbach's Alpha = 0.72 (mobility subtest at 25–42 months) to 0.97 (atypical Positions subtest at 7–12 months)

Test-retest reliability: $r = 0.96$ (mobility) to 0.99 (motor organization, atypical positions)

Decision consistency: 100% (atypical positions), 85–91% (mobility), 94–97% (stability)

Interrater reliability: $r = 0.88$ (motor organization, level c)–0.99 (mobility, motor organization level A, B, and atypical positions)

Standard error of measurement: 0.52 (atypical at 7–12 months) to 1.59 (mobility at 25–42 months)

Construct validity: age-trend analysis indicates that with increasing age, children perform an increasing number of items and master increasingly more difficult items, supporting the developmental basis of item construction

Discriminant validity: mobility, stability, atypical, motor organization, and social-emotional subtests all discriminate children with delays from children without delays

Specificity: 92.6% (mobility), 96.9% (stability), and 98.6% (atypical positions)

Sensitivity: 88.2% (mobility), 80.6% (stability), and 97.2 (atypical positions)

ADMINISTRATION

The primary subtests are administered in the following order: social-emotional, mobility or motor organization, stability, and functional performance. The parents interact with the child following the examiner's instructions. In the mobility subtest, the parent places the child in various positions and the child's sequence of responses are observed and recorded. The motor organization includes 117 items that are administered through play between child and parent. The items of the stability subtest are observed during the administration of the mobility and motor organization subtests. Functional performance is completed by

(*continued*)

CHAPTER 3

(continued)

parental interview. The three clinical subtests are intended to be used by practitioners with advanced knowledge of motor development. They provide information on the quality of a child's movement repertoire. They are particularly helpful for children in whom neuromotor dysfunction is suspected. Scoring varies depending on scale. The five primary subtests yield scaled scores.

TIME REQUIRED

10–20 minutes for infants and 20–40 minutes for toddlers

15 minutes to administer functional performance subtest interview

ADVANTAGES

- Detailed
- Provides visual descriptors
- Parent involvement
- Links function, quality of movement, and skills
- Primarily observation
- Strong psychometric characteristics

LIMITATIONS

- Complicated procedures for recording information
- Can be lengthy initially
- Expensive
- Training tapes would be helpful

ORDERING INFORMATION

Psychological Corporation
19500 Bulverde Road
San Antonio, TX 78259

TRANSDISCIPLINARY PLAY-BASED ASSESSMENT— REVISED (TPBA-R)

Toni W. Linder

PURPOSE

To identify intervention needs, develop intervention plans, and evaluate progress made by children

AGE RANGE

6 months–6 years

AREAS TESTED

Cognitive
Social-emotional
Communication and language
Sensorimotor

PSYCHOMETRIC CHARACTERISTICS

Criterion-referenced
No psychometric information provided in manual

(continued)

(continued)

ADMINISTRATION

Administered by a team consisting of the parents and representatives from various disciplines. The team observes the child during play activities with a play facilitator, the parents, and a peer. Before observation, the family completes a developmental checklist regarding the child's performance at home. This is used to plan the play session. The play session consists of six phases: unstructured facilitation (child leads, facilitator follows and expands), structured facilitation, introduction of peer to observe interaction, unstructured and structured play with parents, unstructured and structured motor play, and snack. Observation worksheets are completed according to test guidelines. Summary sheet describes the child's strengths, rating of abilities, justification of the ratings, and recommendations.

TIME REQUIRED

60–90 minutes

ADVANTAGES

- Can be used with children with disabilities
- Companion curriculum, "Transdisciplinary Play-Based Intervention: Guidelines for Developing a Meaningful Curriculum for Young Children"
- Videotapes available that explain and demonstrate process
- Includes family members in the process
- Nontechnical language facilitates participation of family members
- Information gained is helpful to establish and implement an intervention plan

LIMITATIONS

- Requires team planning
- Initially time-consuming
- Does not provide status of child compared with children of his or her age

ORDERING INFORMATION

Paul H. Brookes Publishing Co.
PO Box 10624
Baltimore, MD 21285-0624

VULPE ASSESSMENT BATTERY-REVISED (VAB-R)
Shirley German Vulpe

PURPOSE

To determine skill performance, strengths and needs, degree of central nervous system functioning, and environmental influence on task performance

AGE RANGE

Children with atypical developmental or functional skills between birth and 6 years

AREAS TESTED

Assessment of basic senses and function: analysis of sensory-motor abilities

Assessment of developmental behavior: developmental skill acquisition

Assessment of the environment: caregiver characteristics and interaction

Performance analysis system

(continued)

(continued)

PSYCHOMETRIC CHARACTERISTICS

Criterion-referenced

Interrater reliability: ICC = 87; percent agreement = 0.88–0.95

Intrarater reliability: r = 0.94

Intrarater reliability of gross motor section: r = 0.87

Concurrent validity of gross motor scales with Peabody Developmental Scales—Gross Motor Scale: Pearson r = 0.97

ADMINISTRATION

Can be administered in whole or in part, individually or in a group by any person familiar with the child or trained in child development. Directions can be modified to meet the needs of the child. Uses familiar toys and equipment; materials do not come with the test manual. Information gathered from multiple sources (observation, caregiver report, chart review, performance evaluation) used to establish the child's typical behavior. The three sections are rated using three methods to analyze the child's skill and processing related to task performance. There is no information on converting raw scores from the Vulpe Performance Analysis to standard scores or age equivalencies. The tasks, however, are arranged in a hierarchal developmental sequence; thus, an age range can be identified for each skill performed.

TIME REQUIRED

Varies depending on the child and strategy of gathering information (observation, interview)

Can be completed over time

ADVANTAGES

- The performance analysis scale (PAS) is designed to be used as a teaching tool
- Operational definitions of PAS are thorough
- Provides task analysis of developmental milestones
- Component skills are cross-referenced across domains
- Administration can be tailored to meet individual needs of children
- No special equipment or materials are needed
- Provides a great deal of descriptive information on task performance and environmental influences that may be helpful in intervention planning

LIMITATIONS

- Packaged in a three-ring binder that breaks easily and is small; pages tear easily
- Poorly organized; difficult to follow text
- Lacks psychometric information
- Little research on how effective the system is in determining small degrees of improvement
- Score sheet requires examiner to fill in items to be tested

ORDERING INFORMATION

Slosson Educational Publications, Inc.
PO Box 280
East Aurora, NY 14052

FUNCTIONAL INDEPENDENCE MEASURE FOR CHILDREN (WEEFIM)

Carl Granger, Susan Braun, Kim Griswood, Nancy Heyer, Margaret McCabe, Michael Msau, and Byron Hamilton

PURPOSE

To determine the severity of a child's disability, the measurement of caregiver assistance needed in the performance of functional activities, and outcomes of rehabilitation

AGE RANGE

Children without disabilities 6 months–8 years

Children with developmental disabilities 6 months–12 years

Children with developmental disabilities and mental ages younger than 7 years

AREAS TESTED

Motor

- Self-care: eating, grooming, bathing, dressing, toileting
- Sphincter control: bladder and bowel management
- Transfers: chair, wheelchair, toilet, tub, shower
- Locomotion: walk/wheelchair/crawl, stairs

Cognitive

- Communication: comprehension, expression
- Social cognition: social interaction, problem-solving, memory

PSYCHOMETRIC CHARACTERISTICS

Criterion-referenced with items selected and modified from the Functional Independence Measure (FIM)

Content validity with PEDI: 0.80–0.97

Test-retest reliability: Pearson r = 0.89 self-care, sphincter control; 97 transfers-locomotion; 0.99 communication-social cognition; 0.99 total

Interrater reliability: Pearson r = 0.87 self care/sphincter; 0.80 transfers-locomotion; 0.96 communication-social cognition; 0.95 total

Equivalence (between parental report and observation): ICC = 0.93 for total score, range = 0.41 (social interaction) to 0.98 (walk/wheelchair/crawl)

ADMINISTRATION

Each subdomain is scored separately either through observation or report on an ordinal rating scale ranging from total assistance to complete independence. A higher total raw score indicates increased independence.

TIME REQUIRED

10–20 minutes to administer if the parent is being interviewed

ADVANTAGES

- Potential to provide continuity between pediatric and adult measures of functional independence
- Ease of administration

(continued)

CHAPTER 3

(continued)
- Facilitates communication among team members regarding a child's functional independence
- Accounts for performance of the activities
- Takes in consideration caregiver assistance
- Training tape available
- Certification process available

LIMITATIONS
- Does not account for environmental modifications that can increase a child's functional independence
- Emphasizes accomplishment of specific daily activities; does not give credit for mastery of components of these activities
- Documentation of caregiver assistance alone may not provide sufficient and specific information to guide clinical decision-making
- Based on an adult view of disability
- Users must agree to use data collection and outcome reporting system

ORDERING INFORMATION
Uniform Data System for Medical Rehabilitation
State University of New York
Research Foundation
82 Farbert Hall SUNY South Campus
Buffalo, NY 14214

CLINICAL OBSERVATIONS

Physical therapists make clinical observations as part of the measurement process. Areas of observation are based on the needs of the child being assessed. Observations have qualitative and quantitative components. Interpretation of these observations are used in conjunction with the child's history and/or standardized test results to assist the therapist in collaborating with the family and child to form an appropriate treatment plan.

Musculoskeletal
Range of Motion
An accurate measurement of joint range of motion (ROM) in infants and toddlers should take the following into consideration:

Lack of consensus regarding joint ROM values and methodology

Variation in reported reliability of goniometric measurements, possibly due to differences among goniometers (size, number system, and material)

Bony landmarks not fully developed and covered by increased fat in infants make it difficult to palpate and line up the goniometer

Edema, pain, adhesions, strength deficits, and muscle hypertrophy can all affect accuracy of measurement

Children Born Full Term
Upper extremities: similar to adults, although elbow extension can be limited as much as 30° in the full-term infant

Lower extremities: substantial variation exists in reported measurements of lower extremity range of motion. There is a tendency for increased amount of flexion at birth for the child born full term because of neural (CNS maturation), mechanical (position), and environmental (interuterine crowding) factors. This flexor bias decreases over time (Table 3-3)

Children Born Preterm

Lack of flexor bias due to lack of interuterine crowding, CNS immaturity, and extensor positioning

Although extensor bias decreases slightly over time, infants born preterm never demonstrate the extreme flexion that is seen in infants born full term (Table 3-4)

Muscle Testing
Manual Muscle Strength Test (MMT)
Infants/Toddlers

Done through observation

Limited to muscle groups

Focus on essential information: estimate through observation of muscle action in antigravity positions—arc of motion against gravity (i.e., assuming hands and knees position, bottom lifting, bringing feet to mouth)

Observe for a symmetric pattern of performance

Observe for a compensating pattern

TABLE 3-3. Average Value of Selected Lower Extremity Range of Motion, Birth through 5 Years: Full-Term Infants

	Central Tendency Values and Range of Reported Values (degrees)						
	Birth	6 weeks	3 months	6 months	1 year	3 year	5 year
Hip extension limitation	34.2	19	7	7	7	7	7
Hip abduction							
In 90° flexion	72.7						
In extension	55.5 (32–91)				59.3	59.3	54.3
Hip adduction	6.4				30.5	30.5	23.8
Hip external rotation							
In flexion	91.9						
In extension	90 (45–137)	48	45	53.1	58	56	38.5
Hip internal rotation							
In flexion	64						
In extension	33 (35–100)	24	26	24	37.5	39	34
Knee extension limitation	17.9 (0–43.3)				5.4	5.4	5.4
Popliteal angle	27 (20–40)		18 (15–30)	10.5 (5–15)	0 / 0		

CHAPTER 3

TABLE 3-4. Average Value of Selected Joint Measurements: Preterm Infants*

	Birth	4 months	8 months	12 months
Hip extension	166.6 (155–175)	161.4 (150–178)	163.1 (120–180)	164.1 (90–180)
Hip abduction (extension)	62.2 (50–90)	61.4 (40–90)	61.1 (35–90)	67.9 (15–90)
Popliteal angle	50.8 (125–180)	144.0 (112–180)	144.1 (117–180)	146 (125–175)
Angle dorsiflexion	127.5 (105–145)	127.7 (101–150)	122.9 (90–160)	118.5 (102–160)
Scarf sign	1.52 cm (0–⁺4 cm)	−0.08 cm (⁻5–⁺4 cm)	.27 cm (⁻4–⁺4 cm)	1.2 cm (1–2 cm)
Elbow extension	178.6 (165–180)	174.5 (160–180)	179.8 (175–180)	180
Wrist extension	98 (95–120)	103.7 (90–135)	100.2	101.2 (90–130)

*Ranges are given in parentheses.

Children

Consider body weight and size when considering level of resistance

Observe for a symmetric pattern of performance

Observe for compensatory movements

Isolated joint actions and specific muscle testing should be limited to children with language development appropriate to follow traditional MMT instructions (approximately 7–10 years of age)

Muscle Power
- Isometric power: ability to hold a position against gravity or known resistance; apply force to muscle in shortened range
- Isotonic power: ability of muscle to move through range with resistance applied throughout
- Eccentric power: ability to resist a force as muscle is lengthened
- Concentric power: ability to resist a force as muscle is shortened
- Repetitive power: ability to produce adequate power for 10 repetitions
- Speed of contraction: ability to adapt quickly throughout range

In young children and/or children with developmental disabilities, power can and should be assessed in functional developmental positions. For example, the squat-to-stand maneuver assesses eccentric control of the gastrocnemius and quadriceps muscle groups when the child moves down into the squat; when rising to a standing position, eccentric control of the hamstrings and concentric control of the quadriceps is assessed. At full upright, concentric control of gluteal muscle group is assessed. Repetitive power can be assessed by asking the child to repeat the squat-to-stand maneuver several times. Asking the child to start and stop at different speeds will assess the speed of contraction.

Isokinetic
Isokinetic testing provides a fixed variable resistance that is totally accommodating throughout the range of motion

Follow instructions provided by manufacturer of the isokinetic testing apparatus used

Minimal amount of normative data available

Effects of age, height, and weight must be taken into consideration

Posture
Torticollis

Observe the infant for asymmetry in supine, prone, and sitting; infants with torticollis typically will laterally flex head to the right and rotate the face and chin to the left

Assess passive and active range of motion of the neck and upper extremities to determine whether limitations and/or contractures are present

Assess motor development to determine influence of torticollis on developmental milestone acquisition

Assess hips for possible dislocation and spinal asymmetry

Scoliosis

A minimal amount of clothing should be worn by the child

Align the child with a plumb line (physical or imaginary)

The child should assume a natural standing posture with feet together

Assess flexibility of the hip: Thomas test

Inquire about functional limitations and/or pain during participation in sports, dancing, or other activities

Observe the position of the head, trunk, hips, and legs from the front, back, and side noting any asymmetries

- Unequal shoulder level
- Scapular prominence
- Uneven waist lines/hip prominence
- Pelvic asymmetry
- Unequal distance between arms and body
- Unequal knee level
- Excessive thoracic kyphosis or lumbar lordosis

Forward bending test

- Sit or kneel behind the child with your eyes level to the waist
- Ask the child to bend forward from the waist until spine is approximately parallel to the floor, knees are straight, and arms are hanging with palms together
- Observe for compensatory unilateral rib hump

Kyphosis

Observe for excessive forward head

Observe for excessive rounding particularly of thorax region

Lordosis

Observe for increased anterior pelvic tilt

Observe for increased hip flexion

Extremity Alignment

Hip dislocation (Fig 3-3)
Ortolani: Examines Hip Reducibility (Return Dislocated Femoral Head Back Into Acetabulum)

Infant supine

Hip and knees in 90° of flexion

Grasp thigh with middle finger over greater trochanter and thumb on medial thigh

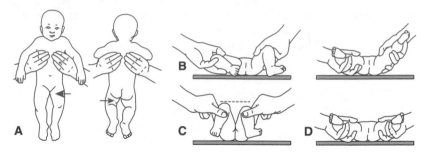

FIGURE 3-3. Signs of hip dislocation. **(A)** Asymmetrical skin folds. **(B)** Limited abduction. **(C)** Apparent shortening of one thigh. **(D)** Examination to elicit relocation or dislocation.

Other hand stabilizes pelvis

Gently lift the thigh to align femoral head and acetabulum and abduct the hip to slide the head over the acetabular rim into the socket

Examiner will feel a definite "clunk"

Barlow: Examines the Ability of the Hip to Dislocate
Infant supine

Knees and hips flexed at 90°

Grasp the thigh with thumb medially over the less trochanter

Other hand stabilizes pelvis

Apply gentle downward pressure while abducting the hip

As femoral head slips over acetabulum rim a subtle "clunk" is felt

Genu recurvatum: knee hyperextension
Genu valgus: knees shifted medially
Genu varus: bowing out of knees
Ankle supination: foot rolls laterally, associated with high arches
Ankle pronation: foot rolls medially
Foot inversion: foot turns in relative to lower leg
Foot eversion: foot turns out relative to lower leg

Biomechanical Analysis
Kinematics

Descriptive analysis of a movement pattern via joint or segment position, joint angles, time, displacement (linear, angular) velocities, and accelerations

Imaging techniques: highly sophisticated motion analysis systems are available, generally in motor control laboratories or gait analysis laboratories; three types are available: cinematography, videography, and optolectric system (Table 3-5)

Kinetics

Represents the pattern of forces that underlie movement

Electromyography

Describes electrical activity of a muscle; interpretation requires corresponding movement analysis

TABLE 3-5. Advantages and Disadvantages of Kinematic Systems

Consideration	Cinematography	Videography	Optoelectric
Ease of use	Somewhat sophisticated	Sophisticated	Very sophisticated
Cost	Moderate to high, except cost of conversion equipment	Moderate, except cost of conversion equipment	Expensive
Frequency	≥64 Hz	60 Hz (USA) <50 Hz (Europe)	≥64 Hz
Encumbrance to movement	Minimal	Minimal	Some
Time to attach	Minimal	Minimal	Moderate
Availability of data for analysis	Film processing and conversion of data high	Instant replay; has capability for instant conversion	Instant conversion
Lighting	Extra lighting required indoors	No extra lighting required for two-dimensional, but may be useful; required for three-dimensional	Extra lighting required
Visual record	Available	Available	Not available unless coupled with video
Laboratory versus naturalistic setting	Both	Both	Laboratory

With permission from Heriza, C. (1993). Kinematic motion analysis. In I. Wilhelm (Ed.), *Physical Therapy Assessment in Early Infancy* (pp. 261). New York: Churchill Livingstone.

Neuromotor
Muscle Tone
Tone can vary in relation to areas of the body or side of the body and may be different in relation to activities and position

Qualitative System
Subjective system: judgment based on resistance to passive movement; on a continuum

Flaccid → decreased resistance to passive movement → normal → initial increase resistance to passive movement and then relaxation to normal as movement continues → consistent resistance throughout movement

Descriptive System (Table 3-6)

Reflexes, Righting Reactions, Automatic Reactions
Primitive reflexes and the righting, automatic, and equilibrium reactions should be assessed by criteria established by the authors of the neuromotor measurement instrument selected (e.g., the NBAS for the full-term neonate, the PDMS-2 for infants and very young children, and the IMS for the preterm infant).

TABLE 3-6. Muscle Tone: Descriptive System

	Hypotonia			Normal	Hypertonia			Intermittent Tone
	Severe	Moderate	Mild	Normal	Mild	Moderate	Severe	Intermittent Tone
Active								
	Inability to resist gravity; lack of cocontraction at proximal joints; limited voluntary movements	Decreased tone primarily in axial muscles and proximal muscles of the extremities; interferes with length of time a posture can be sustained	Decreased tone interferes with axial muscle cocontractions; delays initiation of movement	Quick and immediate postural adjustment during movement; ability to use muscles in synergic and reciprocal patterns for stability and mobility depending on task	Delay in postural adjustment; poor coordination; slowness of movement	Limitation in speed, coordination, variety of movement patterns, and active ROM	Stiffness of muscles in stereotypic patterns; limits active ROM; little or no ability to move against gravity; very limited patterns of movement	Occasional and unpredictable resistance to postural changes alternating with normal adjustment; may have difficulty initiating active movement or sustaining posture
Passive								
	Joint hyperextensibility; no resistance to movement imposed by examiner; full or excessive passive ROM	Mild resistance to movement in distal extremities only; elbow and knee joint hyperextensibility	Mild resistance in proximal and distal segments; full ROM	Body parts resist displacement; momentarily maintain new posture when placed	Resistance to change of posture in part or throughout ROM; poor ability to accommodate to passive movements	Resistance to change of posture throughout the range; limited passive ROM at some joints	ROM limited; examiner unable to overcome resistance of muscle to complete full range	Unpredictable resistance to imposed movements alternating with complete absence of resistance

With permission from Wilson, J. M. (1991). Cerebral palsy. In S. Campbell (Ed.), *Pediatric Neurologic Physical Therapy* (2nd ed., pp. 313). New York: Churchill Livingstone.

Soft Signs

Assessment of soft signs emphasizes how they may affect a child's functional performance on tasks involving movement, perception, and spatial organization

Many of the items examined under soft signs are incorporated into standardized instruments, especially those that focus on sensory processing

Imply a state of immature neurologic function

Items include examination of awkwardness, motor overflow, right-left confusion, mild oculomotor difficulties, primitive postural reflexes observed in positions of stress until 8 or 9 years of age (e.g., ATNR, STNR in the hands-and-knees position)

Vestibular Function and Equilibrium
Postrotary nystagmus test

Prone extension position

Romberg position

Floor ataxia test

Fine Motor Movements
Diadokinesis

Thumb-to-finger touching

Ability to cross midline

Eye-hand coordination

Sensory Testing

Infants: used to determine intact sensation. Apply noxious stimuli (i.e., pin prick) when infant is drowsy and observe for withdrawal, crying, or grimacing. Proceed distal to proximal. Flexor withdrawal response is indicative of spinal cord level response; crying, grimacing, and/or startle responses can help determine level of intact sensation

Children with head trauma: child's response to specific sensory stimuli changes as level of consciousness changes. Stimuli through intact auditory, visual, olfactory, gustatory, and pain pathways evoke a response at all levels of consciousness except at the deepest level of coma (Level V)

- Level I: Child is orientated to time and place and responds to stimuli without delay
- Level II: Specific testing of proprioception; sharp-dull, and two-point discrimination limited by child's cognition and age
- Level III: individualized response to specific stimuli; delay often occurs before response (Table 3-7)
- Level IV: generalized response to any stimuli; response is same regardless of stimuli

Balance

There are clinical tools that can be used in addition to static balance and dynamic balance tasks assessed on standardized measurement batteries

Clinical Test for Sensory Interaction and Balance (CTSIB)

Individual postural sway while standing for a maximum of 30 seconds is observed in each of 6 conditions (Fig 3-4)

Scoring is based on amount of sway and amount of time the individual maintains erect standing; also records changes in perception (dizziness, nausea) and movement strategies used to maintain stability

Most children older than 9 years of age easily maintain stability under all conditions

TABLE 3-7. Localized Response to Sensory Stimuli—Level III

Sensory Tract	Stimulus Examples	Response
Auditory	Voice Bell Hand clapping	Eye opening Looking toward stimulus Turning head toward/away from stimulus
Visual	Threat near eyes Bright object Familiar toy Familiar person	Blinking Focusing and tracking
Olfactory	Ammonia	Grimace or turn away
Gustatory	Sugar Lemon	Smile Grimace
Pain	Squeeze muscle belly Squeeze nail bed, pin prick	Pull extremity away Look toward pain

With permission from Blaskey, J. (1991). Head trauma. In S. Campbell (Ed.), *Pediatric Neurologic Physical Therapy* (2nd ed., pp. 221). New York: Churchill Livingstone.

Abnormal reliance on vision or increase in sway under conditions 3–6 indicates sensory interaction deficit

Functional Reach

While the child stands without assistance, his or her ability to reach forward as far as possible without taking a step is measured (Table 3-8)

Reach scores below critical values may indicate a delay

Gait

Gait can be analyzed with motion analysis systems (Table 3-9)

See Chapter 1 for a description of gait changes throughout early childhood

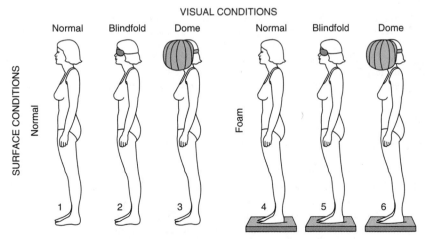

VISUAL CONDITIONS

FIGURE 3-4. Sequence of six conditions for testing the influence of sensory interaction on balance.

TABLE 3-8. Functional Reach Scores Ages 5–15 Years

Age (Years)	Mean Reach (cm)	Critical Reach (cm)
5–6	21.17	16.79
7–8	24.21	20.57
9–10	27.97	25.56
11–12	32.79	29.68
13–15	32.30	29.58

With permission from Donohue, B., Turner, D., & Worell, T. (1994). The use of functional reach as a measurement of balance in typically developing boys and girls ages 5–15 years. *Pediatric Physical Therapy, 6,* 189–193.

Oral-Motor and Feeding
Facial and Intraoral Anatomy

Oral Function
Biting and chewing
Suck-swallow coordination

Endurance

Self-Feeding
Utensil use
Drinking

Oral Motor/Feeding Assessment Scales
Specific tools available to test oral-motor functioning directly; some are described in the instrument section of this chapter and include the following:
Prespeech Assessment Scale (PSAS)
Oral Motor Feeding Rating Scale
Neonatal Oral-Motor Assessment Scale (NOMAS)
Behavioral Assessment Scale of Oral Function in Feeding

Pulmonary Function
Pulmonary Function Tests
Forced vital capacity (FVC)

Peak expiratory flow rate (PEFR)

Forced expiratory volume in 1 second (FEV_1)

Residual volume (RV)

Ratio of FEV to FVC (FEV/FVC)

Functional residual capacity (FRC)

Forced expiratory flow ($FEF_{25\%-75\%}$)

Clinical Observations
Chest
Unmoving: observe shape and symmetry of the thorax; observe for pectus excavatum, funnel chest, pectus carinatum, and scoliosis
Moving: determine respiratory effort; compare right and left thorax for symmetry
Synchrony: compare thoracic and abdominal movement

TABLE 3-9. Motion and Assessment Methods

Type	Description	Advantages and Limitations
Observational gait analysis	Visual evaluation of gait parameters; should include anterior, lateral, and posterior placement of observer relative to moving child	Naturalistic, minimal intrusion on child's spontaneous behavior; can be immediately applied and ongoing; can be used to guide treatment decisions and intervention during treatment session
		Recording of observations by progress note or by communication to child, family, or colleagues; locomotor behavior not documented in a reproducible way for comparison with subsequent evaluations
		More consistent with single than multiple observers; events lasting < $\frac{1}{16}$ seconds or at multiple joints cannot be captured accurately by the human eye
Videotaping or cinematography	Dynamic recording of locomotion using videotape or motion picture camera	Provides documentation of visual gait evaluation which, if carried out in a reproducible manner, can be used for comparison; in conjunction with other gait evaluation techniques, can be a valuable method of recording in a standardized fashion
		If camera placement is not carefully considered in relation to child's position, this may be of little value, especially if each recording session is not performed in a standard fashion; may be useful to record temporal aspects of gait, but degree of error in recording and playback systems is difficult to assess and control for unless timer is incorporated into frames
Digitizing	Method of determining joint angles; can be applied to videotaped data to provide kinematic information on static joint position and changing joint angles; can also be coordinated	Can increase value of videotaped data significantly if joint angle measurements are desired; computer software programs available for this purpose

(continued)

TABLE 3-9. Motion and Assessment Methods (continued)

Type	Description	Advantages and Limitations
	with other types of gait evaluation done in the laboratory; if skin markers are used with good background contrast, automatic tracking of marker positions and digitizing are possible while taping with some systems	following videotaping, although it can be done manually Value and accuracy of digitizing depends on value of videotaped data; camera placement in relation to movement is critical; may require up to three to four cameras
Footprint recording	Many inexpensive approaches, including stepping in water and walking across a firm surface, stepping in powder and walking on continuous paper from a large roll; child can step in ink or paint before walking on paper; paper that is treated to respond to foot placement with a permanent visual display can be purchased (Shutrak or Fuji Prescale)	In conjunction with videotaping can provide comprehensive means of objective gait assessment in treatment setting; can measure step and stride length, base of support, and toe-out or toe-in angle; using a stopwatch, can also measure temporal parameters such as velocity and cadence
Mirrored Plexiglas standing frame or walking surface	Foot contact patterns can be photographed in standing and occasionally during walking	Relatively inexpensive means of recording foot pressure by photography; generally limited to static standing Limited data yield in proportion to equipment expense, although may be useful for guidance in orthotic fabrication and adjustment
Pedobarograph	Means of measuring pressure beneath foot during gait using an elastic mat on top of an edge-lit glass plate; pressure during walking compresses mat onto glass differentially, decreasing reflectivity in proportion to increased pressure; monochrome image under glass processed into color image corresponding to different levels of pressure	Generally available in gait laboratory; data much more elaborate and precise than from other foot contact pressure methods but at considerably greater expense; graphic aspects of data display useful for formal presentation or publication
Force platform or force plate recording	Measures ground reaction forces as ambulator walks over it, providing kinetic data; consists of rigid surface with underlying transducers that measure surface displacement in three axes; ideally mounted flush	Used mainly when ground reaction force data are combined with kinematic information; sources of error include failure to shield system from outside influences and

(continued)

TABLE 3-9. **Motion and Assessment Methods** (continued)

Type	Description	Advantages and Limitations
	with walkway; data collected by microcomputer; force plate data can also be used to evaluate energy changes occurring as center of mass rises and falls	inability of platform to respond accurately when the full foot is not on the platform
Instrumented walkway	Instrumentation is within walkway, not on walker; used to measure timing and placement of foot contact; if used with photoelectric beams, can also measure gait velocity; switch contacts are within walkway itself; or electrical contacts on walker's shoes (requiring cable attachment) close circuit with conductive substance on walkway	Data collection done by microcomputer, but system can be expensive and unreliable because of switch contact malfunction; in-shoe placement of switches may provide similar data at considerably less cost
Electrogoniometry	Direct measurement devices applied to the child; two types of electrogoniometers most often used are potentiometers and flexible strain gauges; provide kinematic data relating joint angles and time, or angular relationships of more than one joint Most commonly used for knee and less often for hip and ankle; trailing wires or cables transmit data to microcomputer	Direct measurement of joint rotation, multiple goniometers can be mounted in several planes in an attempt to provide three-dimensional recording Multiple error sources include invasive nature of recording on child's behavior and difficulty of aligning goniometer with true joint axis in a dynamic situation; even multiple goniometers may not capture degrees of freedom in a joint; digitizing with videotaping or optical kinematic recording may be preferable for most children
Electromyography	Direct measurement of muscle activation patterns, generally used in conjunction with simultaneous recording of other gait parameters; superficial electrodes most commonly used; data collected and integrated by means of microcomputer requiring trailing cable attached to moving child or use of telemetry unit; fine wire or needle electrodes provide more specificity for individual muscle recording but are typically not used for gait analysis, especially in children	Abundant amount of normative EMG data for all age groups provides valuable means for comparison; little value if isolated from time points in gait cycle because it provides information about electrical activity, not mechanical activation; cross-talk among adjacent muscles makes inferences about group activity relatively accurate, but not for individual muscles Potential sources of error: movement, external sources of artifact

(continued)

TABLE 3-9. Motion and Assessment Methods (continued)

Type	Description	Advantages and Limitations
Kinematic systems	Used to record position of body segments, angles of joints, and corresponding velocities and accelerations; several options available: photographic systems or videographic systems with digitizing capability, television/computer systems using reflective markers providing reconstruction of data in three dimensions on television screen, opticoelectric systems using light-emitting diodes as joint markers which are coded by an opticoelectric camera, and opticoelectronic scanners using passive reflective markers that are color-coded to indicate markers positions	Provide abundant opportunities for data collection on multiple joint movements under laboratory-controlled conditions; especially useful for investigative purposes and baseline gait analysis before orthopedic surgery; data collection and integration performed by a microcomputer but still quite labor-intensive; trained personnel essential, full-time engineer often necessary for hardware management; expensive to set up and maintain; intimidating environment for child, may influence performance
Combined kinematic and kinetic motion analysis system system	Provide ability to combine force plate (kinetic) data with kinematic information, allowing limb segment to be evaluated as total mechanical	Most sophisticated of motion analysis systems; very expensive; can be intimidating; multiple sources of breakdown and error
Assessment of energy costs of locomotion	Several methods available: measurement of oxygen consumption and/or carbon dioxide production using a gas measurement and collection system; estimation of energy cost using kinematic data by estimating mass of body parts × distance traveled × acceleration; monitoring heart rate as a function of speed to determine physiologic cost index; and using kinetic data (ground reaction forces) and kinematic data to estimate energy cost with inverse dynamics calculations	Sophisticated method of analysis; requires knowledge of pulmonary function in addition to movement

Retractions: indrawing of thorax during inspiration

General appearance: skeletal abnormalities

Head and Neck

Flaring of the nose, head bobbing, audible sounds: expiratory grunting, color, cyanosis, pallor, plethora

Coughing and Sneezing

Stimulate oral or nasal pharynx to elicit cough or sneeze to determine whether functional

TABLE 3-10. Normal Heart Rate and Blood Pressure Measurements in Children

	Birth–1 Month	Up to 3 Years	Older Than 3 Years
Heart rate (bpm)	120–200	100–180	70–150
Blood Pressure (mm Hg)			
Systolic	60–90	75–130	90–140
Diastolic	30–60	45–90	50–80

Reprinted with permission from Gould, A. (1991). Cardiopulmonary evaluation of the infant, toddler, child, and adolescent. *Pediatric Physical Therapy, 3,* 9–13.

Auscultation
Listen for breath sounds

Strength, Posture, Flexibility, and Endurance
These should also be measured in older children and adolescents

Vital Signs
Heart rate and blood pressure (Table 3-10) as well as respiratory rates (Table 3-11) should be checked

Pain
There are several pain scales available that can be used with children (Table 3-12)

Preseason Screening Evaluation of Adolescent Athletes
Components

Muscle strength	Flexibility
Power	Cardiovascular endurance
Endurance	Joint stability
Speed	Posture
Agility	

Contraindications
There are many contraindications for exercise testing in children (Box 3-2)

TABLE 3-11. Normal Respiratory Rates for Children

Age	Breaths per Minute
Birth–1 month	35–55
Up to 6 years	20–30
6–10 years	15–25
10–16 years	12–30

Reprinted with permission from Gould, A. (1991). Cardiopulmonary evaluation of the infant, toddler, child, and adolescent. *Pediatric Physical Therapy, 3,* 9–13.

TABLE 3-12. Selected Pain Measurement Scales for Children

Self-Report Measures

Oucher scale	5–12 years	100-point vertical scale of 6 photos of children's faces indicating pain intensity
Faces scale	6–8 years	Faces indicating pain intensity
Visual analog scale	5 and above	Child indicates pain intensity on a vertical or horizontal continuum

Behavioral Scales

Children's Hospital of Eastern Ontario Pain Scale (CHEOPS)	Any age	6 observed behaviors (crying, facial expression, verbal complaints, trunk position, touching behavior, and leg position) scored on a 1- to 3-point scale; operational definitions provided
Gauvain-Piquard rating	2–6 years	15 behaviors divided into three subscales: pain, behavior, and psychomotor alterations

Physiologic Methods

Heart rate, EEG
Blood pressure
Respiratory rate
Metabolic rate
Oxygenation $TCPO_2$

BOX 3-2. Contraindications for Exercise Testing in Children

Acute febrile condition

Acute inflammatory cardiac disease (e.g., pericarditis, myocarditis, acute rheumatic heart disease)

Congestive heart failure—uncontrolled

Child with asthma who is dyspneic at rest, or whose FEV or PEF are less than 60% of height

Acute renal disease

Acute hepatitis, during 3 months' onset

Child who has insulin-dependent diabetes who did not take prescribed insulin or who is ketoacidotic

Drug overdose affecting cardiorespiratory response to exercise (e.g., digitalis or quinidine toxicity, salicylism, or antidepressants)

Adapted from the American Heart Association. (1983). American Heart Association Report: Standards for exercise testing in the pediatric age group. In O. Bar-or (Ed.), *Pediatric Sports Medicine for the Practitioner.* New York: Verlag.

Physical Fitness Assessment Scales

Specific tools available to determine level of physical fitness

Physical Best: The AAHPERD Guide to Physical Fitness, Education and Assessment (1989), published by the American Alliance for Health, Physical Education, Recreation and Dance in Reston, Virginia, focuses on health-related fitness

- Aerobic endurance
- Body composition
- Flexibility
- Muscular strength
- Muscular endurance

Intervention

Pediatric physical therapists intervene with children who have a variety of problems affecting their ability to move. Treatment is individualized to meet the unique needs of each child and family. Contemporary physical therapy practice is based on the process of disablement as described in the *Guide to Physical Therapy Practice* (1997). Prevention and wellness strategies are integrated into a comprehensive intervention plan. Intervention focuses on the impact a condition or impairment has on function. This chapter provides a framework for intervention. Treatment strategies and comprehensive treatment goals are described. Treatment protocols are provided for conditions that usually follow protocols, such as some orthopedic conditions. As a rule, however, due to the unique nature of the developing child, the needs and concerns of his or her family, and the complexity of developmental and neuromuscular conditions, treatment strategies must be individualized.

INTERVENTION FOCUS

Although intervention is designed to meet the specific needs of a child, there are four general areas of focus for the therapist. Therapists partner with families and other service providers to support the child in reaching his or her potential by

- Promoting active movement
- Promoting functional skills
- Promoting societal integration
- Preventing impairment

INTERVENTION COMPONENTS

According to the *Guide to Physical Therapy Practice* (1997), physical therapy intervention has three components

- Coordination, communication, documentation
- Patient/client instruction
- Direct intervention

COORDINATION, COMMUNICATION, DOCUMENTATION

Ensures appropriate, coordinated, comprehensive, and cost-effective services

Collaborating with other providers of services, service agencies, and other resources diminishes likelihood of service duplication

Specific Functions of the Pediatric Physical Therapist

- Care management
- Service coordination
- Intervention plans
- Discharge planning

- Care conference
- Referral to other professionals/resources

Communicating With Parents (Box 4-1)
Documentation (see Chapter 6, page 251–255)

PATIENT/CLIENT INSTRUCTION

When appropriate, parents and children should be instructed in activities that reinforce and expand therapeutic goals, objectives, and activities. Therapeutic strategies should be incorporated into naturally occurring activities and routines. Activities should be monitored and adapted on a regular basis.

BOX 4-1. Communicating With Parents

Use correct terms for identifying the diagnosis. When there is more than one term to identify a diagnosis, use the term that is preferred by the parents. Ask the parents their preference and then continue to use it.

Use correct definitions when defining the diagnosis (e.g., Down syndrome is a chromosome disorder). Define terms in concrete ways.

Look up the diagnosis to refresh your memory. In many instances, years pass before some disabilities are seen for the first or second time. Providing false or unsure information can be harmful to the parent and may jeopardize the relationship between the parents and the professional.

Get acquainted with the child. This is a way of showing your interest in the child as a person and not just a disability.

Touch or hold the child and call the child by name as you talk about him or her. By showing an interest in the child's name, you express an interest in the child as an individual.

Discuss the therapeutic plan when both parents are together, if possible.

Call parents by name and use Ms., Mrs., and Mr. as appropriate, unless the parent has given explicit permission to use his or her first name.

Respect parents' needs and feelings about their private space.

Show caring and sympathy. Spend some time with the parent. Be kind and pleasant in your encounters.

Allow parents to express their emotions. Allow them to cry, be sad, or vent anger.

Let parents have positive hope for their child's future when they voice it.

Allow parents to use coping mechanisms that seem to be working for them. Such mechanisms may include their religious beliefs or refusing to accept the diagnosis immediately.

Talk about other siblings or ask about them.

Be sure that parents have a list of available community resources, telephone numbers, and addresses to meet their needs.

Include a parent organization among your list of resources.

Respect culturally based communication styles.

Adapted from Poyder, F. (1995). Better ways (to break news to parents). *Parents Helping Parents,* San Jose, CA.

DIRECT INTERVENTION

Approaches

Remedial

Therapists identify performance deficits, seeking to resolve them by facilitating age-appropriate sensory-motor capabilities

Encourages the attainment of developmental skills and typical movements

Sometimes referred to as the establish or restore approach

Compensation

Compensation minimizes effects of a disability through adaptation of tasks, materials, or the environment

This approach uses assistive technology, adaptive equipment, or other devices to allow a child to perform a skill when he or she is not capable of it or has yet to master it

It is often used with older children with orthopedic or severe neuromotor dysfunction such as spastic quadriplegia, but it is highly recommended to be considered with younger children

Compensation is often used to prevent further impairment or disability, bypassing a barrier to the performance of a desired outcome

Promotion

Use of naturally occurring routines and activities to promote skill development

Often used in community-based activity programs

May be particularly helpful for children with global developmental delays or weakness in performance areas

Prevention

This approach focuses on the prevention of secondary impairments or disabilities in children with known difficulties

Requires therapists to anticipate outcomes and future difficulties

Models

Direct

Therapeutic skills provided directly to a child by a physical therapist or physical therapist assistant under supervision of a physical therapist

Often used to provide intensive remedial intervention but can be used with other approaches

Monitoring

A therapist creates a plan and instructs another team member in its implementation

Therapist is responsible for documentation and ensuring that the plan is appropriately and safely implemented

Increases the likelihood that therapeutic strategies are integrated into naturally occurring activities and routines

Consultation

Therapist provides expertise to another team member to solve a specific problem

Collaborative-consultation is an interactive process involving team members of various disciplines

Three components

• Dynamic interaction among team members
• Respect for each team member

• Belief that consultation will help reach a common goal

Requires ongoing interaction and joint problem-solving

Intervention Techniques

Pediatric physical therapists use a variety of techniques to promote motor function, promote quality and efficiency of motor performance, and prevent impairment. Many of the techniques are similar to those used with adults with physical disabilities, pain, or impairment. The following section provides basic definitions of the techniques commonly used by pediatric physical therapists. It is recognized that there are other techniques being used by therapists; however, it is not possible to describe all techniques. Critical appraisal of the efficacy of each technique is not possible due to the nature of this book. As with other areas of physical therapy, the reader must keep abreast of current research regarding treatment techniques. The techniques are listed in alphabetical order, not in the order of importance.

Physical Handling

Hippotherapy

Incorporates specific therapeutic techniques/strategies while a child is on a horse

Provides multiple sensory inputs (including vestibular, visual, and proprioceptive) to the child

Goals are improved balance, posture, coordination, strength, and flexibility

Appropriate for children with a variety of diagnoses including but not limited to cerebral palsy, muscular dystrophy, spina bifida, and developmental delay

Massage

Involves tactile techniques varying from gentle to vigorous

Used with children with a variety of problems including babies born prematurely

Contraindications

• Infection
• Abnormal body temperature
• Influenza
• Severe upper respiratory infection
• Tuberculosis
• Congenital dysplasia of the hip (CDH)
• Wounds
• Acute illness

Research has shown a variety of benefits, particularly in babies born prematurely

• Improves gastrointestinal functioning
• Improves blood and lymphatic circulation
• Improves weight gain
• Assists in decreasing tactile hypersensitivity
• Promotes parent-infant bonding
• Is calming
• Is comforting
• Improves respiration

Myofascial Release (MFR)

Specific techniques performed by a therapist to release fascial (connective tissue) restrictions

The goal is to change fascial structure, allowing functional change in range of motion

The technique is based on the principle of low load over long duration, with gentle stretch applied to the line of muscle fibers or fascia

Contraindications

- Systemic or localized infection
- Open wounds
- Healing fractures
- Acute inflammation
- Cancer

Precautions

- Osteoporosis
- Hypotonia

Mobilization

Based on the concept that immobility affects all systems necessary to produce movement

Indicated when extraarticular connective tissue abnormally restricts joint motion

General guidelines

- One hand stabilizes the body, while the other hand mobilizes
- Therapist must consider direction, velocity, and amplitude of movement
- No greater than grade III mobilization

Contraindications

- Osteoporosis
- Joint inflammation
- Hypermobility

Neurodevelopmental Treatment (NDT)

Involves direct handling of the child to inhibit abnormal responses and facilitate typical movement patterns

Handling is altered in response to changes in muscle tone and movement patterns

It is designed specifically for young children with cerebral palsy

Sensory Integration (SI) Therapy

Controlled sensory input to help children with sensory processing problems integrate sensations from the body and the environment

Based on three assumptions

- Individuals receive information from their bodies and the environment, process and interpret the information within their central nervous systems, and use the information in a functional manner
- Individuals with problems in sensory processing will have problems in planning and performing motor acts
- Individuals who receive sensory stimulation within a meaningful context will integrate the sensory information, demonstrating more efficient motor skills and adaptive behaviors

Sensory integration equipment is used to engage children actively in sensory stimulation activities in a meaningful, self-directed context (Table 4-1)

Indications

- Tactile defensiveness
- Poor motor planning
- Decreased attending skills
- Inadequate body awareness

TABLE 4-1. Uses of Sensory Integration Equipment

Goal	Equipment	Description
Promote antigravity flexion	Bolster swing	Encourages antigravity flexion or postural balance in sitting
	Flexion disc/swing	Swing with flat disc and center post at right angles to each other
		Holding center post develops flexor muscles
		Varying degrees of difficulty based on amount of support from flexion swing
	Rope ladder	Suspended from ceiling; used to encourage motor planning and improve strength and eye-foot coordination
	Zip swing or flying trapeze	Horizontal glider; also used to increase tolerance to movement
	Hot dog swing Trapeze bar swing Inner tube Vertical bolster	
Promote thoracic extension	Hammock sling swing	Provides support to child in prone to encourage head and thoracic extension
	Scooterboard	Wooden, plastic, or carpet-covered base with four wheels; similar to flat skateboard allowing prone mobility; various sizes and shapes
		Also used to increase upper extremity extensor strength, shoulder forward flexion, head lifting, thoracic extension, and sensory feedback
	Barrel	Lying prone over barrel, child walks his or her hands forward to encourage thoracic extension
Promote gravitational security	Cocoon swing Hammock swing Platform swing Trampoline/bouncing pad	Provides graded movement experiences controlled by child to gradually increase tolerance to movement
Promote balance and equilibrium	Bolster swing	Encourages antigravity flexion or postural balance in sitting
	Hippity-hop ball	Ball with handle that child sits on top of and bounces to move it forward
	Platform swing	Large, flat, square surface providing therapist with large, mobile surface to challenge child's balance and equilibrium reactions

(continued)

TABLE 4-1. **Uses of Sensory Integration Equipment** (continued)		
Goal	Equipment	Description
	T-stool	Small disc with short vertical pole; child sits on it and maintains balance; incorporates upper extremity activities while sitting
Promote proprioceptive feedback	Weighted vest and collars Hippity-hop balls	Advantageous for children with ataxia
Promote tolerance to vestibular stimulation	Sit and spin	Commercially available flat disc that child sits on and turns in circles by turning a center wheel
	Trampoline	
	Bolster swing	
	Foam blocks and crash pad (moon pad)	
	Hammock swing	
	Scooterboard	
Promote motor planning	Rope ladder Barrel	

Techniques used in SI therapy
- Swinging
- Rocking
- Bouncing
- Spinning
- Obstacle courses

Strength Training
Progressive resistive exercises (PREs) are the key to strength development

Strengthening programs should be incorporated into sport activities/programs played by young children and adolescents; these programs should include a warm up and cool down, and exercises should be carried out through a full range of motion; maximum lifts should not be attempted

Strength training should occur 2–3 times a week for short intervals (<30 minutes)

Resistance should be added gradually (1- to 3-lb increments) after proper form is demonstrated

The use of standard PRE protocols may relate to improvement in function in children with a variety of conditions including cerebral palsy and spina bifida

Creativity including the use of the child's own body weight and adaptive equipment will be necessary in strengthening programs for children with disabilities

Caregiver/patient instruction is imperative to prevent injury through incorrect technique, especially when using weights or exercise bands

Research indicates decreased strength in children with cerebral palsy, but only minimal information is available on the effects of strength training

Positioning

Used primarily with children with complex neuromotor dysfunction

Used as strategy to facilitate functional skill

Positions should be changed frequently and appropriately to meet the needs of the activity in which the child is engaged (Table 4-2)

Motor-Based Programs

Conductive Education

Originated in Hungary at the Peto Institute

Appropriate for children with a variety of diagnoses, but primarily those with cerebral palsy

Instructors (conductors) are specially trained and certified

Goal is to promote maximal function through intensive, day-long programming

Uses rhythmic intention and sequenced facilitation to enhance organization and production of intentional movement in educational and life tasks

Movement Opportunities Via Education (MOVE)

Comprehensive, activity-based curriculum for children older than 7 years of age with severe neuromotor dysfunction

Teaches basic functional motor skills including sitting, standing, and walking

Implemented by interdisciplinary team that works on the same set of skills for reinforcement and consistency

Involves the use of specialized equipment that promotes sitting and upright ambulation

Electrical Stimulation

Neuromuscular Stimulation (NMES)

Transcutaneous stimulation of muscle through its motor nerve

Activates motor units by inducing action potentials in the motor nerve

Used to improve strength, improve joint range of motion, facilitate motor learning, and decrease spasticity

Parameters (Table 4-3)

Functional Electrical Stimulation (FES)

Used to increase muscle contractions during functional activity

Can stimulate several muscles to obtain sequential or simultaneous contraction

Useful for individuals with lower motor neuron integrity who are not candidates for tendon transfer

Electrode placement: surface

- Directly over motor point of the targeted muscle
- Connect to portable stimulator

Electrode placement: percutaneous

- Implanted into targeted muscle hypodermically
- Lead wire exit
- Connects to portable stimulator
- Increases accuracy over surface electrode placement

Electrode placement: implanted

- Surgically placed on target muscle or the nerve

TABLE 4-2. Basic Positioning Parameters

	Supine	Prone	Side Lying	Sitting
Pelvis and hips (the pelvis should be in line with the trunk with little rotation)	Hips in 30–90° of flexion	Hips in extension	Hips in flexion	Hips at 90° flexion
	Hips symmetrically abducted 10–20°	Hips symmetrically abducted 10–20°	Hips in 10–20° abduction	Hips symmetrically abducted 10–20°
Trunk (the trunk should be straight)	Shoulders in line with hips	Shoulders in line with hips	Shoulders in line with hips	Shoulders over hips
	Neutral rotation of trunk	Neutral rotation	Slight side bending OK	Not rotated
Head and neck (the head should be in a neutral position)	Facing forward	Facing to one side	Facing forward	Facing forward
	Slight cervical flexion	Slight cervical flexion	Slight cervical flexion	Head evenly on shoulders
Shoulders and arms	Arms fully supported	Arms fully supported	Both arms supported	Arms forward
	Arms forward of trunk	Arms forward of trunk	Lower arm forward	
	Forearms rest on trunk or pillow	Flexion at shoulders	Not lying on point of shoulder	
		Flexion at elbows	Lower arm neutral rotation	
			Upper arm may have 0–40° internal rotation	
Legs and feet	Knees supported in flexion	Knees extended	Knees in flexion	Knees at 90°
	Feet held at 90°	Feet supported at 90°	Feet positioned at 90°	Ankles at 90°
			Pillow between knees	Feet fully supported
				Thighs fully supported

From Ratliffe, K. (1998). *Clinical Pediatric Physical Therapy: A Guide for the Physical Therapy Team* (p. 266). St Louis, MO: Mosby.

TABLE 4-3. NMES: Parameters Used for Various Purposes*

	Motor Learning	Strengthening	Spasticity Reduction	Increasing ROM
Frequency	30–50 (pps)	40–50 pps	30–50 pps	30–50 pps
Intensity	To produce many repetitions of a muscle contraction in at least the fair range	Maximum contraction as tolerated	To elicit tetanic contraction	To elicit a fair grade muscle contraction or that which achieves the target ROM without overstressing the joint
On-off times (or therapist activated)	4:12	10:50	4:12	4:12
Ramps	As tolerated by child	1–5 seconds as tolerated by child	As needed to avoid clonus	Set so that joint makes it through range at appropriate speed; larger joints require longer ramp time as do joints involving spastic muscles
Duration	10–30 minutes	10–15 repetitions	Before therapeutic activities	30 minutes for 60–90 repetitions
Treatment frequency	1–2 times a day, 1–5 times a week	3–5 days per week	As needed	As needed

*Child should be asked to attend to sensation of stimulation.

- Connected to an internal receiver-stimulator
- Used with adolescents, young adults, not growing children

Parameters for specific conditions (Table 4-4)

Sensory Level Electrical Stimulation (SLES)
Daytime use of low-frequency current

Provides sensory feedback on muscle during activity

Used with children with weak muscles and those with difficulty perceiving movement

Contraindicated for children who have surgeries, pacemakers, or skin lesions

Can be used in conjunction with therapeutic electrical stimulation

Therapeutic Electrical Stimulation (TES)
Application of low-frequency electrical current to muscles that are atrophied due to disuse

Purported to stimulate muscle growth

Used with children at least 2 years of age with average growth and muscle atrophy

Contraindicated for children who have surgeries, pacemakers, or skin lesions

TABLE 4-4. Functional Electrical Stimulation (FES) Parameters for Specific Conditions*

	Brachial Plexus Injury	Spina Bifida	General Muscle Stimulation
Frequency	10–50 pps	35 pps	30–50 pps
Pulse width	20–300	347	
Intensity	To produce motor stimulation	To produce motor stimulation	As needed for task
On/off time	5–10:20–60 seconds	8:24 seconds	Therapist activates
Ramp	2–3 seconds	None	0–10 seconds
Duration	20–30 minutes	30 minutes	As needed
Treatment frequency	Daily	Daily	As needed

*Select one to two muscle groups based on weakness and ability to stimulate and change muscle groups as necessary as patient progresses. Most common use is to activate anterior dorsiflexion during gait.

Parameters
- Time: 6–10 hours per day, 6 days per week, during sleeping
- Placement: muscle belly
- Amplitude: child feels sensation but there is no contraction
- Rate: 35 pps
- On/off: 12:12 seconds

Interventions for Selected Conditions

Most children seen by pediatric physical therapists have complex conditions requiring individualized treatment planning based on child- and team-specified outcomes; thus, the use of protocols is not appropriate. However, there are treatments for some conditions that follow a protocol. These are listed when appropriate; otherwise, treatments for symptomatology or impairments (i.e., spasticity) are provided.

Brachial Plexus Injury

Most resolve within few weeks of life

General Intervention Guidelines
ROM
Developmental activities incorporating sensory inputs
Splinting to prevent positional deformities
Tendon transfer surgery if significant nerve damage is present
Teaching compensating strategies and use of assistive devices

Orthopedic Conditions

Congenital Hip Dislocation (CHD)
Physical Therapy
- Improve range of motion of hip flexion, hip abduction, and internal rotation
- External rotation to neutral only

Orthoses

Pavlik harness

- Used with infants 0–9 months of age
- Promotes gradual, dynamic reduction
- Requires reliable/consistent caregiving
- Places child in hip flexion, abduction, and neutral rotation

"A" frame

- Used for children 9 months to 4 years of age who are active and ambulating
- Designed with medial metal uprights connected by a horizontal bar under the groin
- Places hips in abduction and internal rotation, knees in extension, and feet in neutral
- Gait training involves a four-point crutch gait with one crutch in front of the child and one behind

Hip-knee-ankle-foot orthoses (HKAFO)

- Children older than 4 years of age
- The braces are a unilateral double upright long leg brace with a pelvic band
- Hips are placed in abduction and internal rotation

Legg-Calvé-Perthes Disease

Physical Therapy

- Hip range of motion measurements in all planes must be taken carefully and repeatedly
- Emphasis on range of motion of hip in all directions with special attention to internal rotation and abduction
- An orthosis may be needed to maintain the femoral head in contact with the acetabulum
- Teach the child and caregiver methods of donning and doffing the brace and gait training with the orthosis

Orthotic choices

- "A" frame
- Toronto brace
- Petrie cast
- Atlanta or Newington brace

Scoliosis

Surgical Intervention

A rod system is placed from the first thoracic vertebrae to the sacrum to establish normal sagittal plane alignment; postoperative loss of spinal mobility

Physical therapy

- Caregivers are taught lifting techniques to prevent forces on the spine
- Sitting balance, range of motion of the extremities, and strengthening are the primary focus
- Seating systems may need to be adapted after surgery

Torticollis

Physical Therapy

Intervention ideally begins in the first 2–3 months of life

Passive exercises

- Neck rotation to the ipsilateral side with the head in flexion and neutral
- Lateral neck flexion to the contralateral side
- Neck flexion with head in neutral

Positioning

- Encourage looking to the ipsilateral side through environmental adaptations (i.e., turning the crib so that the action is on the uninvolved side)

- Carrying positions that encourage ipsilateral rotation and contralateral rotation or midline position (i.e., carrying the child facing outward to encourage midline positioning of the head and neck)

Active exercises

- Midline activities in supine, prone, sitting, and standing, paying attention to spinal alignment as well
- Rolling toward the ipsilateral side first on a flat surface than up an incline
- Head/body righting activities encouraging contralateral lateral neck and trunk flexion

Orthotics

Several types (Table 4-5)

Spasticity Management

Oral Medications (Table 4-6)

Botulinum Toxin Type A (Botox, Dysport)

Acts presynaptically at nerve terminals to prevent release of acetylcholine with resultant chemical denervation

Procedure

- Injections given to one muscle at a time
- More effective in smaller muscles
- Effect is in injected muscles and possibly adjacent muscle
- Onset of effect is 12–48 hours after injection
- Peak action is 5–10 days
- Duration is 2–4 months
- Injections can be repeated
- Injections can be done at any age
- Good for localized spasticity

Side effects

- Minimal, none reported with normal doses
- Not known how long a child can receive continual doses of Botox

TABLE 4-5. Orthotics Used for Children With Torticollis

Type of Collar	Indications	Construction
Soft	Lateral flexion in all positions	Made from small adult cervical collar with a small area cut out on the contralateral side to allow lateral flexion in that direction
	Inability to fully rotate head to ipsilateral side	
	Poor response to exercise	
	Used to orient child to midline	
Hard	Soft collar no longer effective	Low-temperature plastic
	Poor response to exercise program	Surrounds head and neck, holding them in midline
	Treatment initiated after 6 months of age	Padding placed in ipsilateral side promoting shoulder depression
	Neck extensor muscles and trapezius very tight	

TABLE 4-6. Oral Medications Used in Treatment of Spasticity

Medication	Indication	Side Effects
Benzodiazepines (diazepam [Valium], clonazepam [Klonopin])	Resistance to passive range of motion Hyperreflexia Painful spasms	Sedation, weakness, gastrointestinal symptoms, memory impairments, incoordination, confusion, depression, ataxia
Baclofen (Lioresal)	Spasticity of spinal origin Hyperreflexia Resistance to passive range of motion Painful spasms and clonus	Sedation, weakness, hypotonia, ataxia, confusion, fatigue, nausea, dizziness, lower seizure threshold
Dantrolene sodium (Dantrium)	Resistance to passive range of motion Hyperreflexia Spasms and clonus	Weakness, drowsiness, nausea, diarrhea, lethargy, liver toxicity
Tizanidine (Zanaflex)	Hypertonia and spasm preferentially in spastic muscles To eliminate muscle weakness side effects of other medications Spinal cord injury or multiple sclerosis in persons older than 12 years of age	Dry mouth, dizziness, headache, nausea

Physical therapy
- May be more intensive after injection, with special attention paid to improving range of motion and strength in appropriate muscle groups

Intrathecal Baclofen Pump (ITB)
Similar to γ–aminobutyric acid (GABA), a neurotransmitter believed to produce muscle relaxation
ITB is delivered directly to the spinal cord; thus, muscle relaxation is produced with small amounts of medication thereby reducing side effects
Procedures
- Externally programmable pump is implanted subcutaneously in the abdomen with a catheter placed in the spinal canal
- The pump releases prescribed amount of intrathecal baclofen as instructed by the external programmer
- The pump reservoir holds enough ITB for 1–4 months
Candidates
- Children 4 years of age or older and large enough to accommodate the pump
- Ashworth scale greater than or equal to 3
- Patient/family/caregivers agree on specific, realistic goals and are committed to the process

Risks
- Sedation (overdose can lead to coma)
- Seizures

Selective Dorsal Rhizotomy (SDR)
Used to reduce spasticity in children with cerebral palsy
Transection of dorsal (sensory) rootlets in the spinal cord based on EMG responses

Candidates
Used with two groups of children based on goals

Goal: Facilitate or Maintain Ambulation
- Child 3–6 years of age with spastic diplegia and normal cognition (has also been used with younger children)
- Preambulator, ambulatory with device, or an independent ambulator
- No fixed contractures/deformities or previous orthopedic interventions
- Antigravity muscle strength 4/5
- Family/caregiver committed to procedure and rehabilitation

Goal: Improve Ease of Caregiving
- Child with severely increased muscle tone interfering with caregiving
- Child has nonfixed contractures

General Treatment Considerations
Intense program of intervention: 5 times per week for 6–8 weeks and then 2–3 times per week for 8 weeks to 6 months postoperatively
Strengthening through weight-bearing
Gait training as appropriate

Risks
Sensation loss
Bladder dysfunction if roots lower than S1 transected

Physical Therapy for Child With Goal of Ambulation
Before surgery
- Strengthen: back extensors (thoracic, lumbar), hip extensors, hip abductors, quadriceps, dorsiflexors
- Increase ROM of hip, knee, and ankle if necessary
- Teach postoperative home program
- Review surgery and rehabilitation with parents and child
- Arrange for rental or purchase of postoperative adaptive equipment such as prone stander, wheelchair, posture walker, adaptive chair, and toilet aid
After surgery
First month
- Align pelvis, trunk, and head in sitting: vertical pelvis and thoracic extension
- Increase ROM: thoracic extension, hip extension, abduction, knee extension, dorsiflexion, toe extension
- Strengthen: hip extension, abduction, adductors, quadriceps, hamstrings, all foot and ankle muscles
- Practice weight-bearing
- Develop reciprocal movements in legs
Months 2–4
- Strengthen antigravity control and power
- Strengthen isolated movements in legs

- Prepare feet for weight-bearing: ankle alignment, toe extension, posterior-anterior weight shift
- Strengthen balance reactions
- Gait training: increasing endurance and speed as tolerated

Possible Physical Therapy-Related Problems After SDR Surgery (Table 4-7)

Peripheral Nerve Blocks

Used to reduce activity of the nerve by dissolving myelin sheath and axons

Agents injected into the peripheral nervous system from the nerve root to the motor end-plate

Site selection

- The more proximal the site, the greater the effect and the longer the duration
- Motor point block: injected into the muscle

Agents

- Local anesthetics lasts 1 to several hours
- Effects of phenol/alcohol are reversible, lasting 3–6 months

Injections

- Close proximity to motor end-plate
- General anesthesia
- Electrical stimulation used to locate optimum site
- Can be repeated 4 times

Risks

- Nerve blocks: sensory loss
- Motor point blocks: localized pain

TABLE 4-7. Problems and Possible Solutions After SDR Surgery

Possible Problem	Strategies
Hypotonia	Positioning: chair, prone stander, AFOs
Lumbar laminectomy	Avoid trunk rotation, hip flexion beyond 90°
Weakness	Strengthen hip abductors, extensors, quadriceps in end-range; hamstrings in the midrange, hip abductors, anterior/posterior tibialis, gastrocnemius/soleus muscle throughout the range
Sensory changes (hypersensitivity in feet, anal-genital area, and tops of thighs)	Wear shoes, socks, AFOs Counsel parents and child
Increased ROM	Strengthen muscles in new range all around the joint
Abnormal movement patterns	Relearn new patterns in available range
Lack of trunk rotation	Strengthen trunk rotation: abdominals (especially obliques), thoracic and lumbar spine
Muscle weakness	Specific muscle strengthening, PREs, functional strength training

AFOs, ankle-foot orthoses; *PREs,* progressive resistive exercises.

Age range of children, general goals
- 18–24 months: reduce spasticity
- 30–48 months: improve gait
- Older than 5 years: maintain ROM

Orthopedic Procedures
Muscle Tendon Lengthening (Table 4-8)
Performed to correct a deformity or weakened muscle

Percutaneous Muscle/Tendon Lengthening
To decrease the gamma efferent feedback load by selection of the muscle producing the bulk of this load

Specific muscles within groups such as the hamstring are released while others are left untouched

Physical therapy
- Follow surgeon's recommendation for activity limitation
- Generally, start with active range of motion and then move to passive as healing is completed
- Strengthening and functional skill training

Muscle Transfers

Muscle attachments are moved to another location to change the direction of force production, so that there can be an increase in function

To decrease spasticity, attain a normal alignment, and promote functional skills

Two types
- Recessions: typically, recessions change two joint muscles to a one joint muscle
- True transfers: these involve moving the muscle to a new location, where it will be performing a different action; casting until healing has occurred is required postoperatively

Physical Therapy

Recessions: similar to muscle lengthening

True transfers: intense therapy 2 times a day for the first 3 months with emphasis on motor relearning and functional skills

TABLE 4-8. Common Muscle Groups That Are Lengthened in Children With Cerebral Palsy

Muscle Group	Goal
Achilles	Reduce gastrocnemius contracture
	Improve foot position in a child who toe-walks
Hamstring	Improve knee extension in gait
	Reduce knee flexion contracture
Iliopsoas	Reduce hip flexor contractor and reduce lordosis
Adductors	Reduce scissoring gait
Adductor longus, gracilis, and iliopsoas	Reduce mild hip subluxation
	Hamstring may be lengthened as well to prevent frog-leg or windswept deformity

Hamstring Transfer Protocol
Post operative day 2–4 (discharge on day 4)

- Tilt table (as long as osteotomy has not been performed)
- Out of bed to geri chair

Home rehabilitation

- 4–6 weeks (while in cast) postoperatively
- Continue standing in cast
- Phase 1, (after cast removal)
  - 2 sessions daily
  - Avoid sitting as much as possible during first 4–6 months to avoid adhesions
  - Substitute prone and supine standers for chairs
  - Increase sitting after the child can assume an erect posture easily
  - Stair climbing for reciprocal, disassociated hip movement and strength building
  - Walking exaggerating gait components
- Phase 2
  - Integrate gait components into a more fluid gait with less exaggeration through practice on level surfaces
- Phase 3
  - Higher-level gait functions

Osteotomy

Cutting, removing, or repositioning of bone to enable proper alignment

Common sites in children with neuromotor problems include the hip (derotation) and the tibia

Physical therapy

- Follow surgeon's protocol for weight-bearing and passive range of motion
- Focus on strengthening and gait training

Children in Pain

General Focus
Reduction of pain

Restoration of function

Manage activities of daily life

Strategies
Modalities (Table 4-9)

Ultrasound

- Used with caution, not on epiphyseal plates
- Used with phonophoresis

TENS

Biofeedback

- Auditory, visual, and temperature feedback systems available

Hydrotherapy

Therapeutic Exercise
Complementary Therapies

Relaxation

Massage

TABLE 4-9. **Physical Therapy Modalities for Use in Pain Management**

	Effects	Indications	Contraindications
Ultrasound	Subcutaneous thermal and nonthermal effects	Pain, swelling, scar tissue, adhesions	Over epiphyseal plates
Phonophoresis	Antiinflammatory	Swelling	Over epiphyseal plates
Electrical stimulation	Re-education of muscles	Muscle weakness	Pacemakers
	Blood flow	Swelling	
	Wound healing	Sores	
	Bone growth	Fractures	
TENS	Pain management	Pain	Pacemakers
Biofeedback	Muscle relaxation	Weakness	None
	Muscle re-education	Proprioceptive deficit	
Temperature biofeedback	Warming or cooling of local part	Circulatory	None
Hydrotherapy	Circulation	Cool or hot limb	None
	Cooling or warmth	Hypersensitivity	
	Tactile stimulation		
Therapeutic exercise		Per diagnosis Physician's discretion	

Therapeutic touch

Acupressure

Manual techniques

Infants in the Neonatal Intensive Care Unit (NICU)

General Goals
- Promote developmental organization and physiologic homeostasis
- Minimize postural disorganization
- Promote basic components of movement
- Promote family-centered care

General Considerations

Infants in the NICU are fragile and require intervention by experienced pediatric physical therapists

Interventions are designed to be developmentally appropriate, collaborative, and noninvasive

Assess environment and modify as needed

Identify various equipment attached to infant and ensure that all lines are free and untangled

Assess baseline physiologic status

The infant may only be able to handle one or two types of sensory input at a time; therefore, introduce sensory input slowly

Maintain a collaborative relationship with medical and nursing staff

Be aware of guidelines for appropriate physical therapist practice in the NICU (Sweeney et al., 1999)

Strategies

Positioning

Used to minimize disorganization by providing boundaries, encouraging midline orientation, and discouraging arching and retraction

Handling/Therapeutic Exercise

Used for arousal or calming of infant and promoting components of movements as infant matures

Sensory Interventions and Environmental Adaptations (Table 4-10)

Incorporate Positioning and Handling Into Daily Caregiving

Infant Massage

TABLE 4-10. Sensory Interventions in the NICU and Environmental Adaptations

Sense	Interventions/Adaptations
Lighting	Cover incubators/open cribs with blankets
	Encourage dimming of lights when holding, feeding infant outside of isolette or crib
	Encourage cyclic dimming of the lights to establish normal biological rhythms
Sound	Speak softly, especially when holding an infant
	Do not prepare medications or use top of isolette as a workstation
	Close portholes gently
	Keep monitor alarm volumes down
	Use isolette covers and blankets over open air cribs as buffers to sound
	Place tape players with tapes of maternal heart beat in the isolette, keep volumes low
	Line trash cans to muffle sound of lid closing
Touch	Place infant on gel mattress, eggshell crate, or lamb's wool to eliminate hardness of surface
	Provide boundaries by using bendy bumpers, blankets rolls, diaper rolls, or stuffed animals to assist with positioning
	Provide input with your whole hand versus poking at the infant with one finger
	Move infant slowly and in one movement
	Warm hands before touching infant
	Contain the infant during caregiving procedures
Temperature	If you are going to unswaddle an infant, increase the temperature on the warmer or only unswaddle the upper extremities, rewrap the infant, and then unswaddle the lower extremities; swaddle the infant; place a cap on the head
Vestibular	Developmental positioning to maintain physiologic stability and attempt to self-regulate
	Slow, rocking, up-and-down movements are inhibitory; quicker, side-to-side movements are facilitory

Splinting
- Used to minimize effects of contractures or positional deformities
- Can incorporate taping

Hydrotherapy
Used with medically stable infants to decrease tone, decrease irritability, and increase ROM
Incorporates gentle handling to promote full body relaxation

Kangaroo Care
Skin-to-skin contact providing naturalistic thermal, auditory, proprioceptive, and vestibular input

Feeding
Factors Affecting Feeding Success
A variety of factors influence feeding success (Table 4-11)

Optimal Oral Feeding Technique
Alert baby in enface position, head elevated 45–60°

Flexed position with extremities contained, chin slightly flexed

Proper nipple selection (Table 4-12)

Gradually insert nipple, use tongue as base of support, and provide cheek support (Table 4-13)

Equipment Seen in the NICU
There are many types of equipment seen in the NICU (Table 4-14)

Equipment Used During Treatment (Table 4-15)

Used to assist therapist during a treatment session

May provide biomechanical support or assist child in controlling a specific movement

TABLE 4-11. **Factors Affecting Feeding Success**

Factor	Characteristics
Infant behavior	State
	Endurance
	Age
	Motor skill development
Medical complications	Cardiac
	Respiratory
	Metabolic
	Neurologic deficits
	Extreme prematurity
	Musculoskeletal, i.e., cleft lip/palate
Environment	Stimulation level
	Caregiving technique
	Prolonged feeding time
Timing	Readiness for oral feeding optimally at 36 weeks
	Oral reflexes present at 32 weeks

TABLE 4-12. Nipple Selection Guidelines

Suck Style	Flow Rate	Nipple
Slow feeder	High	SMA Orthodontic
Weak sucker		SMA Enfamil Preemie
Low endurance		NUK
Fast feeder	Low	Enfamil Standard
Decreased coordination of suck-swallow-breath		Ross Standard
Strong suck		
Even paced	Medium	SMA Standard
		Ross Preemie
		Enfamil Natural
		SMA Preemie

Adapted from Wolf, L. S., & Glass, R. P. (1992). *Feeding and Swallowing Disorders in Infants.* San Antonio, TX: Therapy Skill Builders.

Encourages active participation of the child during treatment

Provides variety to activities

General considerations

- Be aware of safety
- Maintain variety to interest child
- Train other caregivers in appropriate, safe use of equipment and precautions to be taken
- All equipment (especially mobile surfaces) requires practice by therapists to control surface and to handle child

TABLE 4-13. Intervention With Nipple

Problem Area	Recommended Nipple Type
Tongue	
Retraction	Round
Flat, hypotonic	Firm
Lacks central groove	Long
Protrusion/thrusting	Long
Lip position/movement	
Poor lip seal	Narrow base
Mouth	Standard
Small in size	Shorter
Hypersensitive gag	Partially insert
Strength of suck	
Weak	Soft
Strong	Firm

TABLE 4-14. Equipment Commonly Seen in the NICU

Equipment	Description
Radiant	Mattress on an adjustable tabletop covered by a radiant heat source; provides open space for tubes and equipment and easy access to the infant
Incubator	Enclosed unit of transparent material providing a heated and humidified environment; access to infant through side portholes
Thermal shield	Plexiglas dome placed over the trunk and legs of an infant in an incubator to reduce radiant heat loss
Oxygen hood	Plexiglas hood that fits over the infant's head to control oxygen and humidification delivery
Mechanical ventilators: pressure ventilator	Delivers positive-pressure ventilation; pressure-limited with volume delivered dependent on the stiffness of the lung
Volume ventilator	Delivers positive-pressure ventilation; volume-limited delivering same tidal volume with each breath
Negative-pressure ventilator	Ventilator that creates a relative negative pressure around the thorax and abdomen, thereby assisting ventilation without an endotracheal tube; difficult to use in infants weighing less than 1500 g
Nasal and nasopharyngeal prongs	System for providing continuous positive airway pressure (CPAP) consisting of nasal prongs of varying lengths and adaptor to pressure-source tubing
Resuscitator	Usually a self-inflating bag with a reservoir (so high concentrations of oxygen may be delivered at a rapid rate) attached to an oxygen flowmeter and a pressure manometer
ECG, heart rate, respiratory rate, and blood pressure monitor (cardiorespirograph)	Usually one unit will display one or more vital signs on oscilloscope and digital display; high and low limits may be set, and alarm sounds when limits are exceeded
Transcutaneous oxygen (Tc PO_2) monitor	Noninvasive method of monitoring partial pressure of oxygen from arterialized capillaries through the skin
Intravenous infusion pump	Pumps intravenous fluids and transpyloric feedings at a specific rate; pump has alarm system and capacity to monitor volume delivered, obstruction of flow, and other parameters
Neonatal vital signs monitor	Measures mean blood pressure and mean heart rate from plastic blood pressure cuff; values are digitally displayed on monitor
Pulse oximeter	Measures peripheral oxygen saturation and pulse from a light sensor secured to the infant's skin; values are digitally displayed on the monitor; some models have continuous recording of values on strip charts

TABLE 4-15. Equipment Used During Treatment

Equipment Type	Comments
Ball/bolsters/rolls	Provides moving surface to facilitate postural adjustments and balance reactions
	Depending on speed of movement, can be relaxing or stimulating
	Consider properties when treatment planning (sizes, colors, textures, and shape) as properties may affect child's interest, enjoyment, and treatment success
	Bolsters can be used for positioning, dynamic sitting activities, lateral balance activities, or range of motion activities, including runner's lunge
Bench	Adjustable height; used to facilitate cruising and transitions (floor to sit and sit to stand)
Dynamic bench, Theradapt	On rocking legs to provide mobile treatment surface
	Assist in encouraging equilibrium reaction
Crawler	Provides support to child's trunk in quadruped, facilitating forward propulsion
Educubes	Chairs that are not supportive or adjustable
	Adaptable to two seating levels
	Can be used as a table
Scooterboard	Wooden, plastic, or carpet-covered base with four wheels; similar to flat skateboard, allowing prone mobility
	Used to increase upper extremity extensor strength, shoulder forward flexion, thoracic extension, head lifting, and sensory feedback
	Various sizes and shapes
Standing poles	Two vertical poles that child holds onto to promote upright posture and balance
	May be used to initiate ambulation
"T" stools	Chair with one leg to challenge child's sitting balance
Tilt board	Provides mobile surface for child to respond adaptively to displacement
Dycem	Piece of rubberized plastic that can be placed under equipment to prevent slipping
	Good to put under plates to prevent sliding while child is eating
	Can place on seat to prevent slippage

Developmentally Appropriate Practice (DAP)

Children with developmental disorders often have multiple difficulties in areas such as communication, attention, and behavior. Providing consistent developmentally appropriate interaction will assist in promoting age-appropriate behavior.

General Guidelines for DAP

Be patient and supportive
Set and enforce reasonable, age and developmentally appropriate limits and expectations
Provide directions and instructions slowly and simply; break down tasks as needed
Make sure child is attentively listening to the directions
Maintain consistency and structure
Provide child with choices from activities and on motions
Allow child time to practice so that information can be processed
Incorporate other children into treatment to promote socialization
Incorporate therapeutic strategies with typical childhood activities

Behavior Management

Intervention with children with disabilities and special health care needs can be stressful and frustrating for the child. Many children with developmental disabilities have difficulty adjusting to transitions, making needs known, sustaining attention, and following directions. Incorporating positive behavior management into programming increases the likelihood that a child will cooperate and actively participate in treatment.

Accept and Respect Children's Feelings

Listen quietly and attentively
Acknowledge feelings
Give feelings a name: "That sounds frustrating"

Instead of Punishment

Express your feelings strongly without attacking
State your expectations; this is very important
Give the child a choice
Problem-solve with the child

Use Positive Reinforcement

Notice positive attributes and actions and let child know that you have noticed

Ignore Inappropriate Behavior

Ignoring may be difficult initially, as behavior may worsen before improving
Ignoring is not the strategy of choice if the child's problem behavior places his/her or
    others' safety in jeopardy or may damage property

Prevent Inappropriate Behavior

Give hugs	Offer encouragement
Anticipate trouble	Clarify messages
Give gentle reminders	Overlook small annoyances
Redirect	Ignore provocations
Give praise and compliments	Point out natural or logical consequences

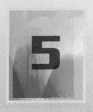

Assistive Technology

Britta Battaile, MHS, PT, PCS

A s defined in the Technology-Related Assistance for Individuals with Disabilities Act ("Tech Act") of 1988–PL199-407, assistive technology (AT) includes "any item, piece of equipment, or product system, whether acquired commercially off the shelf, modified, or customized, that is used to increase, maintain, or improve functional capabilities of (people) with disabilities." AT encompasses mobility devices, positioning aids, prosthetics, orthotics, adaptive toys and games, simple switches, computer switches, access and applications, augmentative/alternative communication, environmental accessibility, medical technology, and also items that improve the general comfort of a person with disabilities. AT devices can be divided into high-tech and low-tech categories, but in essence include anything that promotes a person's access to and participation in the life that he or she wants to lead. This chapter emphasizes AT devices that are used by children with disabilities to influence and improve their functional abilities. Throughout the chapter examples of commonly used and available products are cited. This does not constitute an endorsement of these products. The decision to buy a certain type of product must be made according to the individual needs of the child and his or her family.

▓ FACTORS TO CONSIDER WHEN CHOOSING AN AT DEVICE

Child and family priorities, concerns, and desired outcomes should be included in decision-making

Decisions should be made within a team framework, including input from all appropriate rehabilitation team members (family members, child, occupational therapy, physical therapy, speech therapy, educators, physicians, durable medical equipment professionals, orthotists, and rehabilitation engineers)

Decision-making process can be lengthy and complicated

Questions to pose during decision-making (Box 5-1)

▓ DEVICES FOR MOBILITY

WALKERS

Factors for consideration

- Lower extremity weight-bearing and supported standing skills
- Upper extremity weight-bearing and grasping skills
- Deformities in the extremities and/or trunk
- Upright balance
- Efficiency and speed of supported gait
- Areas of the body in need of support

> **BOX 5-1. Decision-Making Queries**
>
> What is the desired functional goal?
> What are the child's physical and cognitive abilities?
> What is the child's activity level?
> What are the child's endurance and balance capabilities?
> What are the child's visual and perceptual skills?
> What is the level of safety awareness?
> In which environments will this assistive technology device be used?
> In which activities will the child want to participate?
> What might enhance the child's age-appropriate peer interactions?
> What are the psychosocial effects of the equipment?
> What is the safety parameter of the equipment?
> What are the aesthetics of the equipment?
> How much growth and/or adjustability is built into the device?
> What are the costs and funding options?
> What are training and maintenance requirements?

Anterior Walkers

Bar in front (Fig. 5-1)

Used with children who need to support themselves while in some degree of hip flexion or who tend to hyperextend during gait or lose their balance backward

Encourages upper extremity weight-bearing and forward bending

Posterior Walkers

Bar in back (Fig. 5-2)

Often used to encourage upright posture/trunk extension in user

Allows user to move in close to tables, shelves, and people, as there is no anterior bar

Most common type of walker used by pediatric patients

Accessories/Options Available for Anterior and Posterior Walkers

Forearm supports with straps: allow advancement with weight-bearing on forearms and enables those who do not easily maintain grasp to use regular walker (Fig. 5-1)

Pelvic guides for stabilization

Swing-away seats for children with low endurance

Various types of adjustable handles

Baskets or pouches for carrying items

Wheels, swivel casters, or standard tips may be attached to front and/or back legs to influence speed and ease of use depending on the skills and needs of the user

Grade aids to prevent rolling backward on inclines

Large width for the child who walks with a wide base of support

Extra length to prevent tipping

Most fold to some degree for storage/transport

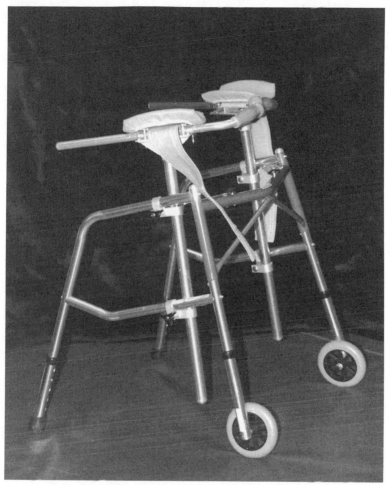

FIGURE 5-1. Anterior walker with front casters and forearm supports.

Support Walkers

Offer substantial support to the child's trunk and/or lower extremities

Usually include a seat for the child to sit on during use

Typically do not encourage fully upright (hips extended) stepping

Gait Trainers

Very sturdy, wheeled walkers that offer any combination of upper extremity, trunk, and perineal support for children who have great difficulty walking but have the ability to reciprocally step with the legs (Fig. 5-3)

Supports can be removed as the child's strength and skills improve

Frequently used to encourage basic ambulation, whether for functional or therapeutic purposes (psychological, bone density, or cardiopulmonary exercise benefits)

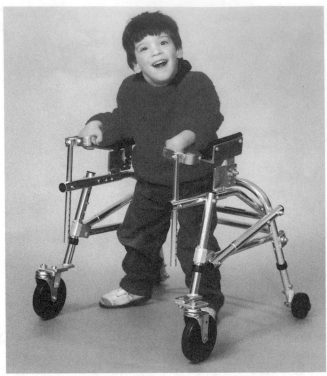

FIGURE 5-2. **Posterior Walker (Posture Control Walker by Kaye Products).**
Reprinted with permission from Kaye Products, Inc.

Locked wheel kits are available to limit sideways movement of the gait trainer, allowing
   only linear, anterior movement

Parapodia

Standing brace similar to a hip-knee-ankle-foot orthosis (HKAFO) that allows some stepping via circumduction (pivot base) or swiveling (swivel base)

May support development of child's self-image and permit some independent maneuver-
   ing in small spaces, but may not be particularly functional or energy-efficient

Used most by children with spina bifida who have significant lower extremity weakness/
   paralysis

Swivel Walkers

Allow advancement in upright via a type of swiveling movement

Not particularly functional due to slow pace and high energy demands

Hands-Free Walkers

User advances device with trunk, pelvis, and lower extremities; upper extremities are
   free

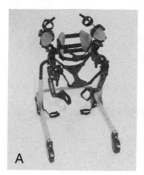 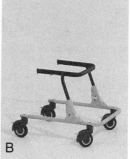

A   B

FIGURE 5-3. Gait trainer with and without accessories. Reprinted with permission from Rifton Equipment.

CRUTCHES AND CANES

Often used in conjunction with lower leg orthoses and are frequently a bridge between us-ing a walker and taking independent steps

Forearm Crutches
Forearm cuffs and hand grips allow significant weight-bearing on the upper extremities

Canes
Single-Footed Canes
Choice of hand grips to suit user's comfort needs and skills
Can be used unilaterally or bilaterally depending on needs
Require better balance than crutches

Quad Canes
Cane with four-prong base of support for increased stability compared with single-footed cane

Accessories for Crutches/Canes
Special-order crutch tips decrease chances of slipping and improve handling on wet floors
Wrist loops to enable user to free up hands for use while simultaneously keeping hold of device
Forearm supports allow weight-bearing between wrist and elbow, holding elbow in a po-sition of approximately 90° of flexion; distribute weight over larger area for improved comfort and control; allow crutch and cane use for those with limited elbow extension

■ DEVICES FOR WHEELED MOBILITY

WHEELCHAIRS
Considerations
• User's lifestyle/environmental needs
• Upper extremity skills
• Strength and endurance

CHAPTER 5

- Cognitive skills
- Visual and perceptual skills
- Head and trunk control
- Deformities that may need to be accommodated
- Transfer method
- Benefit of transition between sitting and supported standing in wheelchair device (as this is an option for increased versatility)
- Transportation needs; availability of vehicle with tie-down system to secure wheelchair
- Independent or dependent use
- Most suitable propulsion method: manual (user's hands on wheels or passive pushing) or battery-powered (via use of a joystick, switch, breath control, or other system)
- Most suitable wheelchair base type
- Most suitable seating system
- Ease of interfacing with other AT devices
- Weight of chair

Wheelchair Base Systems
Manual Wheelchairs

Propelled by advancement of the wheels by the user's upper extremities or passively by someone pushing it

One-arm drive models available

Front-wheel drive models also available; require less shoulder excursion for propulsion

Fold best for storage

Many manufacturers offer transport-ready options for manual bases

Stroller-based manual wheelchair types are often preferred by caregivers of younger children

Optional motorized component is available that converts a manual chair to a power system; decreased frame stability makes this less terrain-versatile

Powered Mobility Systems (Motorized Wheelchairs)

A functional control mechanism for the user to command stopping, going, steering, and speed is required. Common functional control options include joy sticks, toggle switches, simple push buttons, breath control activation, oral keypads, and wafer boards that allow up to four choices of directions and are programmable to meet specific needs of each child. Activation of a functional control mechanism may be via the user's mouth, head, shoulder, elbow, hand(s), thigh, knee, foot, or any other body part or singular muscle that affords consistent and appropriate motor control.

Attendant controls are available for training and safety purposes (steering, stopping, and reversing as well as speed control)

More energy-efficient means of mobility for children who have difficulty propelling a manual wheelchair

Allow the child to keep up with his or her peers

Increase child's sense of environmental control and independence

Good for indoor and outdoor use/all types of terrain

Can accommodate any type of seating system or control mechanism

Substantially heavier than nonpowered chairs; limited portability

Much less compact for storage

Require more care (battery recharging)

Require appropriate cognitive skills to learn control

Seat-to-floor height usually higher than manual wheelchairs

Standard system has large rear wheels

Modular system has four small wheels; sits low to ground; front-, rear-, and all-wheel drive options affect turning radius and stability

Types of Seating Systems

Standard: upright seat with seat-to-back angle fixed at 90°

Reclining: allows reclining to 180° (fully flat position); seat-to-floor height varies

Tilt-in-space: allows angular positioning of seat (fixed at 90° seat-to-back angle) within the wheelchair for individualized comfort and function; used by children who have difficulty holding their head up in upright; may support respiratory efforts (Fig. 5-4)

Linear (Planar) Seating Systems

Use generic, flat supports for postural alignment

For children who have no fixed deformities

Considerable adjustability for growth

Least costly

Contoured (Modular) Seats

Provide standard contouring of appropriate areas (such as low back, hips, and thighs) to support sitting posture

Frequently used by children who need significant support or those with developing or established spinal or other structural deformities

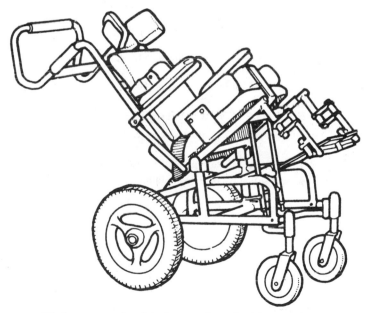

FIGURE 5-4. Tilt-in-space wheelchair. Reprinted with permission from Mark L. Batshaw, MD.

Better pressure relief than linear system

Require frequent adjustments for growth

Custom-Molded Seating Systems

Highly contoured and individualized

Usually for children with complex positioning needs or those who require the snuggest support available for greatest alignment, function, and accommodation of deformities

Can assist in controlling abnormal posturing

Can be designed to alleviate pressure areas and help prevent pressure sores

Limited adjustability and growth accommodation

Most expensive system type

Accessories for All Seating Systems

Headrests: for support, positioning, or transport safety

Trunk supports: harness systems, H straps, lateral supports (fixed or swing-away)

Shoulder retractor straps or protractor pads

Lap belts: for safety and maintenance of pelvic alignment for proper positioning

Lateral or medial supports at the thighs for adduction/abduction positioning

Anti-thrust seats: contoured to prevent loss of appropriate sitting position due to tendency to extend hips

Footrests, straps, and shoe holders: for lower extremity alignment and comfort

Arm supports: for upper extremity positioning and weight-bearing

Trays: wooden, clear acrylic, or polycarbonate

Wedges to correct asymmetric pelvic heights

Lumbar pads or cushions

Wheelchair Seating Measurement Guidelines (Table 5-1)

Troubleshooting/Guidelines for Proper Seating (Table 5-2)

MOTORIZED SCOOTERS/THREE WHEELERS

Powered mobility with seat that may rotate to side for easy transfers; handlebars mounted on central tiller

Seat generally higher than standard seating, requiring specific transferring skills

Child must have adequate sitting balance due to limited postural support

Large turning radius

Child needs appropriate upper extremity control and grip strength to move handlebars and operate forward/reverse modes

NONMOTORIZED SCOOTERS

Prone Scooters

Prone boards (Fig. 5-5)

Allow the child to propel by pushing on the ground with the hands

Often used for mobility after surgery or for those who are cannot bear weight on the lower extremities

TABLE 5-1. Guidelines for Seating Measurements

Measurement	Technique	Special Considerations
Seat width	With braces on, the greater of width across hips or across thighs plus 2–4 inches to allow for growth	For lateral thigh guards on the seat, add 3 inches For abduction pommel or medial thigh supports, add 3 inches
Seat depth	Measure from rear of buttocks to inside bend of each knee (in case of leg length discrepancy) and subtract 1–1.5 inches	If using adjustable-depth hardware, add the amount of the available adjustment to total depth (e.g., if child measures 12 inches, should be sitting at depth of 11 inches and have 2 inches of growth; order hardware with 13-inch depth)
Back height	Measure from underside of buttocks to (1) axillae, (2) top of shoulders, and (3) top of head on both sides	Height should be to axillae for child who will self-propel chair and does not require anterior chest support Height should be to top of shoulders if child will require anterior chest support and headrest If using seat cushion, add half the thickness of the cushion to the measurement for height
Chest width	Measure across chest 1 inch below axillae	Chest width is the minimal distance needed between lateral trunk supports
Chest depth	Measure the depth of chest 1 inch below axillae	Chest depth is the minimal length needed for lateral trunk support pads (if using planar pads) If using curved or contoured lateral support pads, add at least 1 inch to depth measurement
Footrest height	With the child wearing shoes and braces (if indicated), measure the bottom of the thigh to the bottom of the heel with ankle at 90° surface	If using seat cushion, subtract half the thickness of the cushion The footrest must clear at least 2 inches above the floor surface If footrest angle is 90°, the footrest must clear the height of the front caster

Adapted with permission from Kurtz, L., Dowirk, P., Levy, S., & Batshaw, M. (Eds.). (1996). *Handbook of Developmental Disabilities* (p. 297). Gaithersburg, MD: Aspen.

CHAPTER 5

TABLE 5-2. Guidelines and Troubleshooting for Proper Seating

	Optimal Position	Common Problems	Possible Solutions
Head/Neck	Facing forward in midline; able to rotate freely to either side; neck in neutral	Head tilt to one side; head flexed forward; head extended back; forward head posture; swallowing or respiratory difficulties	Check pelvic and trunk positioning; check position and support of shoulder girdle; try different head supports; consider visual issues; consider gravity-assisted reclined positioning
Shoulders	Symmetric, level; no rotation, elevation, or depression; no scapular protraction or retraction	One side elevated or rotated forward or back; scapular protraction or retraction	Use H-strap harness or single sling shoulder straps; protractor pads at scapulae and retractors with posterior head support; check general trunk positioning
Upper extremities	Resting comfortably on lap, armrests, or tray at level of the elbows	Tray or armrest height inappropriate (usually too low); adduction or abduction of upper extremities; retraction of upper extremities (sometimes wedged in between tray and chair); chafing of armpits	Adjust tray; possibly tilt tray up; check lateral trunk supports and elbow stops. Ensure two-finger space between lateral supports and armpits
Trunk/spine	Midline, not leaning to either side; appropriate thoracic and lumbar curves	Trunk leans to one side; kyphosis; scoliotic posturing	Adjust trunk straps; have seating insert accommodate for static deformity; use lumbar support; check trunk harness system for proper fit; adjust lateral trunk supports
Low back/ pelvis/hips	Slight anterior tilt; Symmetric right and left sides; seated all the way back in chair; equal weight-bearing on both ischial tuberosities; hip flexion at 90° or slightly more flexed	Excessive anterior tilt; posterior tilt; one hip higher; one side of pelvis rotated forward or back; pelvis tilted to one side; hips too flexed, extended	Position hips in some degree of flexion to remediate anterior tilt; make sure child is seated all the way back in seat; confirm appropriate seat depth with seat belt across hips (below anterior superior iliac spine with downward and backward pull); ensure that footrests are at *(continued)*

TABLE 5-2. Guidelines and Troubleshooting for Proper Seating (continued)

	Optimal Position	Common Problems	Possible Solutions
			appropriate height; check hamstring length, as extreme tightness may pull pelvis posteriorly; add lift under hip, if necessary to achieve symmetric heights; check seat-to-back angle; consider anti-thrust seat
Thighs	In neutral or slight abduction for comfort; neutral rotation; in full contact with seat until shortly before popliteal areas	Thighs adducted and internally rotated; thighs not fully supported by seat; windswept deformity	Use appropriately adjusted medial and lateral supports; ensure proper width of seat; adjust seat length; accommodate leg length discrepancy, if present; adjust footrest height
Knees	90° of flexion	Front of seat chafes back of knees; top of knees bump against bottom of tray	Shorten seat depth; adjust tray height compatible with upper extremity needs; undercut seat to accommodate hamstring shortening and extend footrests posteriorly
Ankles/feet	Resting comfortably on footrests at 90° or in slight dorsiflexion	Turning in or out of feet; pronation of feet; contractures	Use stabilization straps on footrests; have child wear orthoses; use shoe holders; consider angle-adjustable footrests

Seated Scooters

Low-to-the-ground, go-cart style with large wheels at the sides (Fig. 5-6)

Propelled by the upper extremities

Frequently a child's first mobility device

Often used by children who cannot crawl efficiently or as a prewheelchair training device

MOBILE STANDERS

Intended for upright mobility; user-propelled

Assist the child in maintaining a standing position while allowing mobility and enabling access to the environment (sinks, tables) and peer-level height

Some designed to allow transitioning between standing and sitting

CHAPTER 5

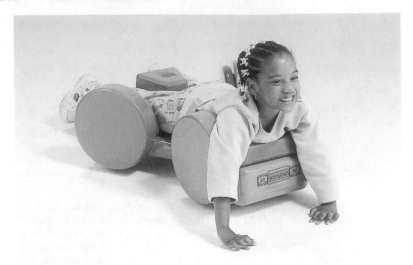

FIGURE 5-5. Prone board (JettMobile by Tumble Forms). Reprinted with permission from Sammons Preston. JettMobile is a trademark of Sammons Preston.

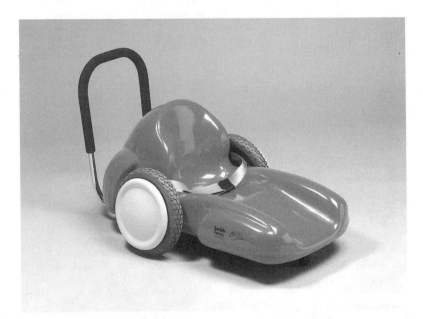

FIGURE 5-6. Seated scooter (Ready Racer by Tumble Forms). Reprinted with permission from Sammons Preston.

STROLLERS

Considerations
- Weight and portability
- Storage and ease of transport
- Aesthetics
- Postural control offered

Commercially Available

Can be used until child outgrows them

May be used in combination with adaptive seating insert to secure better positioning for the child

Specialized Strollers

Resemble mainstream strollers (Fig. 5-7)

Allow for taller, larger, and heavier riders (up to 125 lb)

Examples: Convaid Cruiser and Maclaren Models

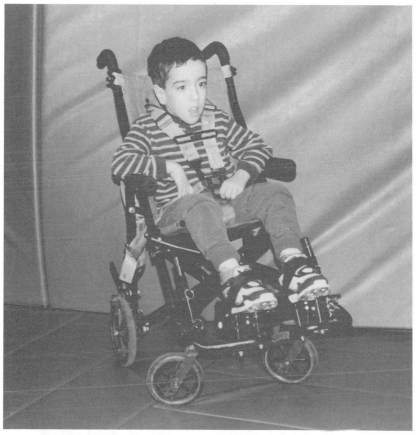

FIGURE 5-7. Specialized stroller.

Accessories

Lateral head and trunk supports

Trunk harnesses or strapping support systems

Hip abduction pommels

Foot plates

Foot/ankle straps

Trays

ADDITIONAL DEVICES USED FOR MOBILITY AND OTHER PHYSICAL TASKS

Motorized toy vehicles: may be good option for promoting mobility, control, and interaction with peers

Crawlers: wheeled devices that suspend or support the trunk of the child in an all-fours position; permit use of upper and lower extremities in a crawling fashion

ORTHOSES

Orthoses are custom-made or custom-fitted mechanical devices designed to improve orthopedic alignment of and support to joints to improve function, promote proper growth and development, and modify muscle tone

Should be designed and made by individuals with experience, expertise, and specific training in pediatric biomechanics and fabrication of orthoses

Balance between degree of control and degree of restriction that any orthotic device provides is delicate

Orthoses can limit overlengthening and assist in preventing tightening of muscles

Many muscles affected by these devices are not significantly activated during use of the device and are therefore prone to disuse atrophy

LOWER EXTREMITY ORTHOSES

Table 5-3 lists the most common lower extremity orthoses (Figs. 5-8–5-10)

UPPER EXTREMITY SPLINTS

Provide support to hand, wrist, fingers, and/or elbow to improve function and to assist in increasing or maintaining functional range of motion

The following are a selection of splint types available

Static Splints

Maintain one or more joints in appropriate alignment

May affect function because of immobilization factor

Made of soft, flexible, or rigid materials

Spasticity-Reduction Splints

Maintain wrist, finger, and thumb extension and finger abduction

Assist in reducing flexor tone in the wrist and hand

Finger Abduction Splints

Maintain fingers in abduction and aid in extension

TABLE 5-3. Lower Extremity Orthoses

Type of Device	Description	Purpose(s)
Heel cup	Plastic support around the heel	Provides minimal medial/lateral stability of heel/ankle in cases of mild instability or pronation
Shoe insert	Plastic and/or foam in-shoe pad that extends along sole of foot; contoured for heel, arch, and ball of foot/toes	Provides mild arch support and proprioceptive input in cases of mild pronation
Inframalleolar orthosis (IMO)	High- or low-temperature plastic; extends from back of foot to front of foot (ball or toes) at level below malleoli	Heel stabilizer with interior posting (such as medial arch support); permits ankle motion in all planes
Supramalleolar orthosis (SMO) (Fig. 5-8)	Plastic; extends from back of foot to front of foot (ball or toes) above level of malleoli	Heel stabilizer with interior posting (such as medial arch support); supports neutral position of the subtalar joint (STJ); permits dorsiflexion and plantarflexion, but limits lateral motion
Ankle-foot orthosis (AFO) Nonarticulating (solid-ankle) (Fig. 5-9) Articulating (hinged) With anterior tibial shell (floor reaction)	Plastic; extends from subfibular head level to underneath foot to ball of foot or toes; anterior shell is also made of plastic and fits on top of AFO	Supports neutral STJ and lower leg-to-foot alignment Solid-ankle design locks ankle in neutral (90°) or in slightly more flexion to assist in preventing knee hyperextension; offers most support of any lower leg orthotic; does not permit tibial advancement. Hinged design allows some dorsi-flexion (and sometimes plantar-flexion), but in a fashion that is unlike natural triplanar motion at the ankle; because of restriction of true ankle motion, may contribute to medial knee ligament laxity in crawling or kneeling. AFO with anterior shell used to assist in achieving full knee extension during gait in cases of significant crouching
Knee-ankle-foot orthosis (KAFO)	Extends from above knee to bottom of foot	Used for standing or ambulation by children with significant lower extremity weakness, such as in myelomeningocele; knee joint may be fixed in some degree of flexion (0–5°) or articulating to allow active flexion
Hip-knee-ankle-foot orthosis	Extends from hip/pelvic level to bottom of foot; includes pelvic	Used for standing and walking in children with significant hip and

(continued)

CHAPTER 5

TABLE 5-3. Lower Extremity Orthoses (continued)

(HKAFO)	band; allows knee flexion or locking into extension	lower extremity weakness
Reciprocating gait orthosis (RGO)	HKAFO with molded body jacket to incorporate trunk; allows knee flexion or locking into extension, cable system	Allows reciprocal gait by children with myelomeningocele or spinal cord injuries; knees may be locked in extension or allow flexion; stepping is initiated by lateral weight shift
Isocentric brace	Similar to RGO, but with less support at thighs, ballbearing system	Same as for RGO, but may be easier for some children to operate
Standing, walking, and sitting hip (SWASH) orthosis (Fig. 5-10)	Consists of pelvic band, thigh cuffs, and steel connectors	Prevents excessive hip adduction and internal rotation in sitting, standing, and walking; theoretically assists in maintaining proper lower extremity/pelvic alignment for improved joint congruity
Twisters	Pelvic band with two straps or cables to attach to shoes or AFOs	Counter excessive internal or external rotation of lower extremities during gait
Spinal (trunk) orthotics Corset Thoracolumbar-sacral orthotic (TLSO)	Various soft and firm materials; surround trunk and extend to pelvic level	Support and/or correct alignment of trunk and rib cage in cases of significant weakness or flexible asymmetry as in scoliosis; can improve postural comfort as well as respiratory, speech, head control, and upper extremity skills; corset used in cases with more easily correctable postural needs; TLSO used in cases when more significant support/correction is needed

FIGURE 5-8. Supramalleolar orthosis (SMO).

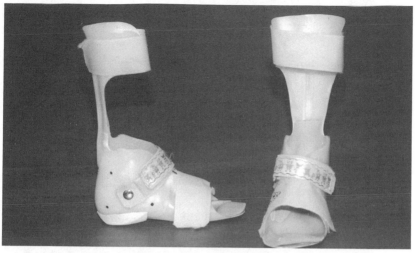

FIGURE 5-9. Ankle-foot orthosis (AFO): nonarticulating solid-ankle.

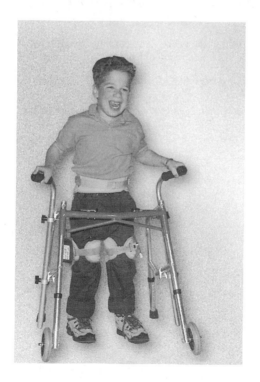

FIGURE 5-10. Standing, walking, and sitting hip (SWASH) orthosis. Reprinted with permission from CAMP Healthcare.

CHAPTER 5

Semidynamic Splints

Allow freedom of movement for some segments while immobilizing others

Cock-Up Splints

Support wrist and palm; fingers are free to move

Thumb loops

Made of soft material such as Neoprene

Hold the metacarpal of the thumb in abduction and extension

Assist in reducing ulnar deviation during functional use of the wrist and hand

Weight-Bearing Hand Splint

Used to maintain the upper extremity in an aligned weight-bearing position to assist in therapeutic activities and performing transitions

Dynamic Splints

Have moving parts that assist in improving alignment and range of motion

Orthokinetic Wrist Splints

Consist of a cone placed in the hand which exerts pressure on the wrist and hand flexors

Forearm shell exerts pressure on forearm flexors

Mackinnon Splints

Wooden dowel placed in the palm of the hand to stretch intrinsic flexors; secured with strap and plastic piece on dorsum of hand

"J" Splints (Dynamic Wrist and Arch Support With Thumb in Opposing Position)

Use palmar bar that wraps around thumb in a fashion resembling letter "J"

Use dynamic forces to maintain wrist in alignment and place pressure on hand flexors to reduce effect of flexor tone

Dynasplints

Bracing system that provides constant tension and can be adjusted to increase range of motion

Can be used at various joints

Expensive

Care is complex

CERVICAL BRACES

Support the head and neck in midline for improved alignment and stability

Commercially Available

Used by children with poor ability to hold head upright or those with torticollis; made of soft material such as foam

Custom-Made

Soft and/or hard materials

May encompass shoulders, jaw, and occiput

■ POSITIONING AIDS

Promote function

Provide the user with support, stability, and improved alignment

Offer access to upright positioning

May influence participation in activities

Available for any functional position: on the floor, in sitting, and in standing

FLOOR-BASED POSITIONING DEVICES

Multipiece Floor Positioners

Offer many options for supported positioning in prone, supine, side-lying, and sitting (Fig. 5-11)

Various sizes available to accommodate all children

Numerous adjustable and interchangeable parts, including tray for play with toys or eating and props for prone-on-elbows play

Infant Seats

Made of soft foam (Fig. 5-12)

Can be used independently on the floor or on a surface with optional floor sitter base (and optional wheeled platform), or in strollers, wheelchairs, or therapeutic swings

Enable bilateral hand use

Allow age-appropriate developmental positions that may promote peer interaction

May be tilted to almost any angle

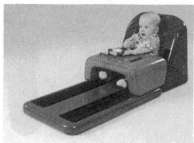
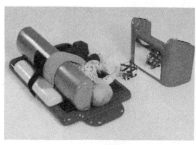
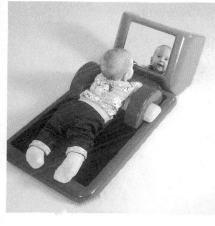

FIGURE 5-11. Multi-piece floor positioner (Tadpole by Tumble Forms). Reprinted with permission from Sammons Preston. Tumble Forms is a trademark of Sammons Preston.

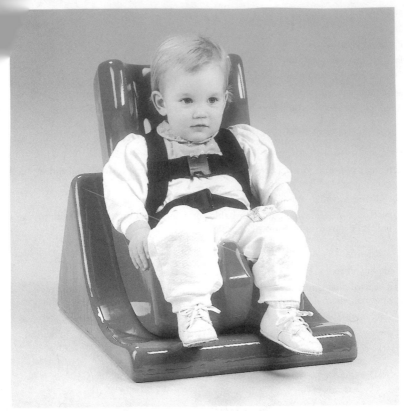

FIGURE 5-12. Infant seat with base (Feeder Seat by Tumble Forms). Reprinted with permission from Sammons Preston. Tumble Forms is a trademark of Sammons Preston.

Are used mostly for infants because they do not support optimal hip or spinal positions

Side-lyers
Allow midline upper extremity use with head and trunk in neutral

Promote weight-bearing or propping on the upper extremities

Legs can be separated by an abduction pad

STATIONARY SEATING AIDS
A child will routinely sit in at least three types of chairs throughout a day: one for eating, another for educational pursuits, and another for recreational times

Pelvis must be all the way back in the chair and should be maintained there in a stable manner in all seats

Proper sitting support and posture constitute a key factor in head, visual, and upper extremity control

Some special-order chairs are available with stroller bases

Commercially Available Seating
High Chairs
Wooden, Step-Ladder–Type Chairs
Allow different heights for seat, feet, and backrest
Come with a seat belt
Optional anterior safety bar at waist level for use with younger children
Easily used at a conventional table
Highly adjustable

Bean Bags
Offer nonspecific propping support
Beware of suffocation hazards

Regular Classroom Chair
With simple belt or trunk strap added

Computer Ergonomic Chairs
Child basically kneels on chair, weight-bearing on shins
Posture while using the chair characterized by anterior pelvic tilt and upright head/neck
Can improve spinal extension and head/neck alignment
May accentuate lordosis
Should only be used by children with relatively good upper body control and no significant lordosis

Special-Order Seating Systems
Posture Chair by TherAdapt
Also allows sitting while supported on weight-bearing knees (Fig. 5-13)

Corner Chairs
Designed for snug, lateral trunk support
Assist in keeping shoulder girdle forward, head in midline, hips at 90°
Optional tray
May sit on floor so that child long sits or off the floor allowing for 90/90/90 positioning

Bolster Chairs
Consist of wooden base that contain a horizontally placed, padded, vinyl-covered bolster that the child straddles for sitting
Assist in keeping the hips abducted and encourage low back extension

Stroller-Base Option Chairs
Covered foam with footrests, headrests, and adjustable tray
Optional stroller base
Example: Carrie Seat by Tumble Forms

Wooden Chairs
Solid wooden chair base with padding, footrests, and tray options
Provides basic sitting support, allowing 70° to 90°/90°/90° positioning
Can be used as a base for custom-made seating inserts
Example: Kinder Chair by Rifton

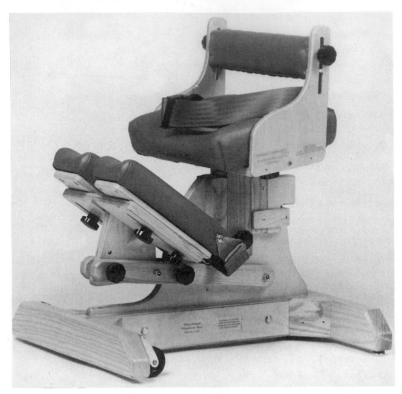

FIGURE 5-13. **Posture Chair.** Reprinted with permission from TherAdapt Products, Inc.

Cube Chairs
Allow 90°/90°/90° positioning
Seating option for children with good, unassisted sitting posture

Benches
Height-adjustable (Fig. 5-14)
Optional attachable pelvic and knee positioning aids

Custom-Made Seating Devices
More expensive; used for children with need for significant support

STANDERS
Enable upright positioning
Promote lower extremity weight-bearing, peer interaction, free upper extremity use, improved head control, midline orientation, and improvement of several physiologic functions (kidney, bowel, digestion)
Benefit bone growth and hip joint development
Can help prevent some contractures, such as hip and knee flexion

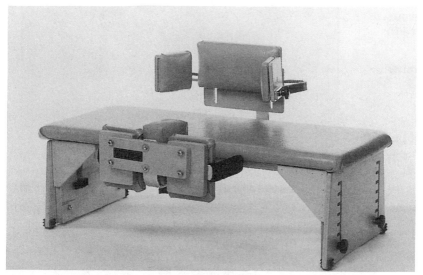

FIGURE 5-14. Bench with positioning aids. Reprinted with permission from Kaye Products, Inc.

Positively influence respiration and sound production

Posture of the user in the stander is vital to the user's functioning

Symmetry, midline orientation, and stable support of key areas such as trunk, hips, knees, and feet are necessary

Trays are available

May be stationary, wheeled (by self or another person), or stationary with wheeled base for transportability between locations; include brakes for safety

Standing Boxes

Trunk-height, four-sided wooden box with tray

User may assume inappropriate lower extremity postures such as hip internal rotation, flexion, and adduction, and knee flexion

Parapodia are similar (see description under Devices for Mobility)

Upright Adjustable Standers

Usually have adjustable fabric straps or firmer support surfaces at trunk, hips, and knees, with weight-bearing surface under the feet

Used by children who can maintain relatively good supported standing posture but who cannot stand entirely unassisted

Often used by children with myelomeningocele

Some offer hip spica options

Supine Standers

Used by children who have difficulties keeping head up for functional lengths of time or who cannot tolerate full weight-bearing on the lower extremities (Fig. 5 15)

Many possible angles of inclination

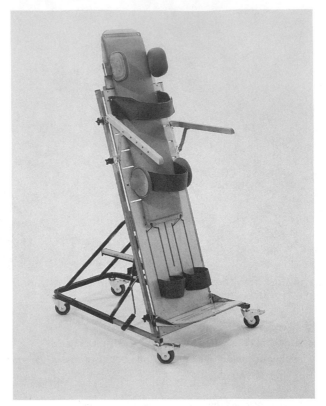

FIGURE 5-15. Supine stander. Reprinted with permission from Rifton Equipment.

Prone Standers

Used by children who cannot maintain upright standing well enough or those who may benefit from practicing head lifting against gravity (Fig. 5-16)

Many possible angles of inclination

All-Position Standers

Allow positioning in prone, supine, or upright

Knee Standers

Support child in a tall kneeling position

Allow upright positioning for those who cannot bear weight appropriately through extended knees or on the feet

Require significant head and trunk control

Patella should be protected from direct weight-bearing

May be uncomfortable for extended periods

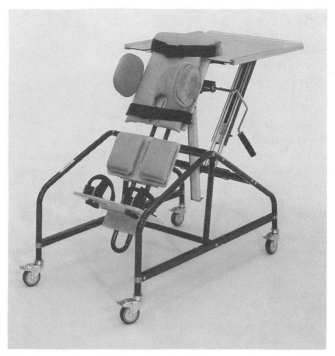

FIGURE 5-16. Prone stander. Reprinted with permission from Rifton Equipment.

■ SELF-CARE AIDS

BATH CHAIRS

Made of fully immersible PVC tubing or stainless steel for the frame and nylon netting for the seat

Seat belts included for safety and positioning

Offer lateral head supports, trunk harnesses, and thigh positioning assists

Can be used in the bathtub, at poolside, or at the beach

SHOWER CHAIRS

Used by older children who can sit unsupported and safely but cannot stand independently for significant periods

Allow hands-free showering and drying off

Optional transfer sections to move in or out over the tub's edge

TOILETING CHAIRS

Offer the following options: high back supports for stability, seat belts, trunk and thigh positioning supports, arm rests, and upper body rests in the form of anterior shelves

GRAB BARS

Can be attached to bathroom walls

Offer safety and support for transfers and maintenance of positions in shower, bath, and while using the toilet

Provide support for washing, toweling off, and dressing

FEEDING AIDS

Adapted utensils: shape, size, handles

High-rim bowls: deter spillage and make loading of utensils easier

Nonslip materials: "anchor" items for easier pick-up and help prevent spills

Cups with special features: weighted bottoms, spouts, handles, cut-out rims

TRANSPORTATION AIDS

VESTS

Can be used with regular seat belts for older children who need extra support

CAR SEATS

Special-order seats with optional head supports, trunk harnesses, low back supports, and thigh abduction assists

Can accommodate children and teenagers who weigh up to 170 lbs

Special seats available for children in hip spica casts

MISCELLANEOUS AIDS

PRESSURE-DISTRIBUTING CUSHIONS

Relieve sitting pressure on the ischial tuberosities

NONSLIP MATERIALS

Can be placed under dishes during meals, under toys or communication devices, or on chairs or bicycle seats to prevent slipping

AIR (PNEUMATIC) SPLINTS

Inflatable splints for extremity joints

Allow positioning in extension when not possible actively

WEIGHTED VESTS

Fabric vests with varying amounts of weight inserted (Fig. 5-17)

Intended to improve proximal stability and sensory awareness

KNEE SKIS

Designed to prevent W-sitting (sitting in a pseudokneeling position characterized by hip flexion with significant internal rotation at the hip; with or without hip abduction)

LIFTS FOR TRANSFERRING

Styles available include those that lift child only or child in a wheelchair

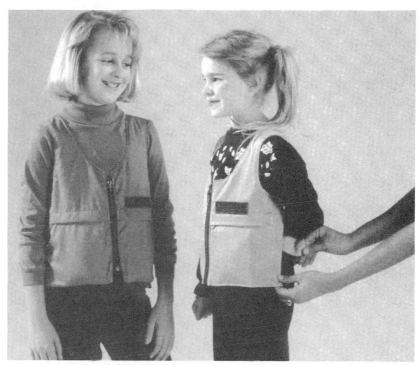

FIGURE 5-17. Weighted vests. Reprinted with permission from Southpaw Enterprises, Inc.

■ ADAPTIVE RECREATIONAL EQUIPMENT

TOYS AND GAMES

Commercially available, battery-operated toys (such as vehicles, animated plush toys, and fans) may be adapted to enable activation by special switches of many types [see Access Methods for Alternative/Augmentative Communication Devices (and Adapted Toys) below]

Adaptive busy boxes with many sensory features and various switches

Game pieces of commercially available games may be adapted for easier grasping, as may items such as paint brushes, crayons, colored pencils, and knobs of puzzles

Adaptive devices for rolling die or using spinners

Toys that are particularly stimulating to the tactile, vibratory, auditory, and visual senses

Adapted rocking horse that sports adjustable seat with positioning supports and straps as well as solid handrails rather than two hand grips

BICYCLES AND TRICYCLES

Commercially available bicycles and tricycles may be adapted with accessories such as back rests, seat belts, foot pedal straps or shoe cuffs, thigh abduction pommels, and upright handlebars that are easier to grasp for some children

Special-order adaptive bicycles come with various supports for trunk, pelvis/hips, and feet;
    may include training wheels for added support; are usually sturdier than commercially
    available bicycles of the same size

Adaptive tricycles also provide numerous adaptive features (Fig. 5-18)

SPORTS EQUIPMENT

Bowling: ramps specially designed for ball release for crutch, walker, or wheelchair users

Ball play: beeper balls that signal to blind players when the ball is approaching

Skiing: specialized equipment to allow skiing in a seated position

Tennis/basketball: sports wheelchairs that are light-weight, compact, and highly maneu-
    verable

Ice skating: push-along, walker-type supports made of PVC tubing

PLAYGROUND DESIGN/EQUIPMENT

Numerous accessible parking spaces

Wheelchair-, crutch-, and walker-friendly flooring that helps protect children in case of
    falls

Wheelchair-width and -height jungle gyms and monkey bars

Ramps for access to jungle gyms

Special swing seats with supportive backs, sides, and seat belts; accommodate large chil-
    dren as well

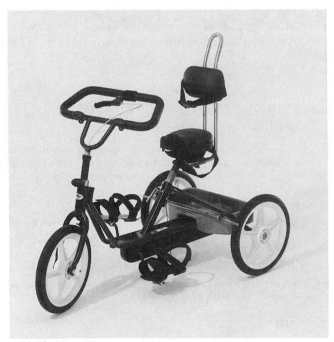

FIGURE 5-18. Adapted tricycle. Reprinted with permission from Rifton
Equipment.

ARCHITECTURAL ACCESSIBILITY

Ramps, door width, door opening mechanisms

Stair climbers allow a child who uses crutches or a walker or fatigues excessively with stair walking to ascend/descend stairs in a seated position; require assistant to activate and guide device

Stair wheelchair lifts allow child in wheelchair to ascend/descend stairs in own wheelchair without having to transfer; lift is installed in staircase

ENVIRONMENTAL MODIFICATIONS AND CONTROLS

Assisted listening devices: TTDs, amplification systems

Ultrasonic transmitters, AC power line control, radio frequency, infrared, and lasers are options for environmental control of things such as light switches, radios, CD players, and televisions

ALTERNATIVE/AUGMENTATIVE COMMUNICATION (AAC) DEVICES

Considerations

- Motor capabilities of child for accessing various devices; which specific body part or muscle will be used to activate the equipment
- Cognitive skills of child: cause and effect, attention
- Vision and hearing skills
- Language and literacy skills; language selection (PicSyms, alphabet, words) most appropriate for the user

COMMUNICATION DEVICES

Electronic output devices (examples: the Wolf, SpeakEasy, and various "talker" and "communicator" devices)

Communication boards and vests

Picture boards

Visual scanners

Clock-style communicators

Specialized computer systems

Access Methods for Alternative/Augmentative Communication Devices (and Adapted Toys)

Each child should be given repeated opportunities over time to try different types of access methods to find the best personal method (or methods)

Access methods may involve use of adapted switches or alternative input devices representing, among others, the following modes of activation

- Pressure- and touch-activated
- Voice-activated
- Movement-, neuro- or specific muscle-activated
- Respiratory-controlled

- Visual scanners
- Light- or head-pointing
- Joystick, toggle, button, and plate switches
- Tilt, roller, pulling, and gripping switches
- Adapted keyboard or mouse

▓ MEDICAL EQUIPMENT TECHNOLOGY

Incubators, warmers, thermal shields

Oxygen hoods and tanks

Monitors: oxygen, blood pressure, ECG, respiratory rate

Ventilators

Intravenous pumps: fluids, feedings

Feeding tubes

Pacemakers

Catheters

Cerebrospinal fluid (CSF) shunts

Tracheostomies

Ostomy bags

Speaking valves

Administrative Issues

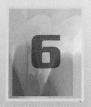

E ffective service delivery and documentation are significant concerns for providers of physical therapy. Physical therapy for infants and children is provided in a variety of environments such as hospitals, public and private educational settings, rehabilitation centers, and private homes. Within these environments, there are often various levels of care based on the seriousness of the illness, purpose of the agency providing the service, needs of the family, and accessibility of service provision. In the past 40 years there has been a gradual shift in the way individuals with disabilities are served. In 1960, children with disabilities were institutionalized and professional care providers assumed the role of custodian. Currently there is an emphasis on including children with disabilities in every aspect of life. Providing services in natural environments, that is, environments in which children without disabilities go to school, to play, to be part of society, is considered the best practice. This chapter reviews the philosophical, legislative, and regulatory issues influencing service delivery, describes various service delivery environments, and presents information on the documentation systems often used when providing physical therapy to children with disabilities within this contemporary system of care (Fig. 6-1).

PHILOSOPHY

Pediatric physical therapy is grounded on six major premises guiding the design of service delivery and interventions

- Family
- First 3 years
- Children are active learners
- Intervention evolves
- External factors
- Cultural competence

FAMILY

The family is the constant in the child's life

Intervention must involve the family at all levels of decision-making

Physical therapists must develop a collaborative relationship with the family (Box 6-1)

FIRST 3 YEARS

The first 3 years of life are critical in the development of a child

The interaction between the child and the environment during this time lays the foundation for future communication, cognition, social relationships, and adaptive performance

CHILDREN ARE ACTIVE LEARNERS

A child's needs and interests must be taken into account when designing intervention and service delivery

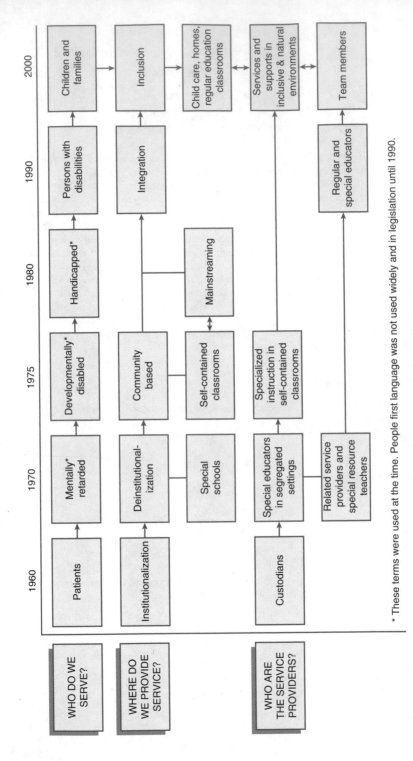

FIGURE 6-1. Paradigm shifts in service provision for children with developmental disabilities.

> ## BOX 6-1. Key Elements of Family-Centered Care
>
> Recognizing that the family is the constant in a child's life, whereas the service systems and personnel within those systems fluctuate
>
> Facilitating parent/professional collaboration at all levels of health care
>
>   Care of the child
>
>   Program development, implementation, and evaluation
>
>   Policy formation
>
> Honoring the racial, ethnic, cultural, and socioeconomic diversity of families
>
> Recognizing family strengths and individuality and respecting different methods of coping
>
> Sharing complete and unbiased information with parents on a continuing basis and in a supportive manner
>
> Encouraging and facilitating family-to-family support and networking
>
> Understanding and incorporating the developmental needs of infants, children, and adolescents and their families into health-care systems
>
> Implementing comprehensive policies and programs that provide emotional and financial support to meet the needs of families
>
> Designing accessible care systems that are flexible, culturally competent, and responsive to family-identified needs
>
> Source: National Center for Family Centered Care, Association for the Care of Children's Health, Bethesda, MD 20814.

Participation by the child and his or her family is necessary within treatment sessions and for decision-making regarding service delivery

INTERVENTION EVOLVES

Intervention is most successful when begun as soon as possible and when the child and family are available to participate actively

Intervention will evolve over time to meet the changing needs of the child and family

EXTERNAL FACTORS

External factors, even if temporary, can influence the development of a child

These factors, which include the child's family, culture, environment, and the social system, must be accounted for when designing intervention

CULTURAL COMPETENCE

A set of congruent behaviors, attitudes, and policies that comes together in a system, agency, or among professionals and enables that system, agency, or those professionals to work effectively in cross-cultural situations

The word "culture" is used because it implies the integrated patterns of human behavior including thoughts, communications, actions, customs, beliefs, values, and institutions of racial, ethnic, religious, or social groups

Competence implies having the capacity to function within a context of culturally integrated patterns of human behavior as defined by a particular cultural group (Box 6-2)

CHAPTER 6

BOX 6-2. Values and Principles Integral to Providing Culturally Competent Services and Supports

The family as defined by each culture is the primary system of support

Individuals and families make different choices based on cultural forces; these forces must be considered if services are to be helpful

The system must sanction and in some cases mandate the incorporation of cultural knowledge into policy-making and practice

Cultural competence involves working in conjunction with natural, informal support and helping networks within culturally diverse communities

Cultural competence seeks to identify and understand the needs and help-seeking behaviors of individuals and families; cultural competence seeks to design and implement services that are tailored or matched to the unique needs of individuals, children, and families

Cultural competence involves determining an individual or family's cultural identity and levels of acculturation and assimilation to be helpful

Practice is driven by culturally preferred choices, not by culturally blind or culturally free interventions

An agency staffing pattern that reflects the make up of the population within the geographic locale helps ensure effective services

Cultural competence embraces the principles of equal access and nondiscriminatory practices in service delivery

---

▪ LEGISLATION (TABLE 6-1)

EDUCATION (TABLE 6-2)

Individuals with Disabilities Education Act (IDEA)

Describes the requirements of special education and early intervention services to children with disabilities (Table 6-3)

Three categories of service requirements are described in the law and subsequent regulations

Special Education Services: Part B

Services provided to children 6–21 years of age

Requires that all states provide a free and appropriate public education (FAPE) for all children with disabilities as described under IDEA

Each child's education follows the plan developed by the team and documented in the individualized education program (IEP)

Physical therapy is a related service and as such is provided to assist with and in support of the IEP

Children should receive appropriate services in the least restrictive environment (LRE)

Preschool Services: Section 619 of Part B

Services provided to children 3 years of age through 5

Requires a specific transition plan be established for children at age 5.5 to prepare for Part B, school age services

TABLE 6-1. Federal Legislation Affecting Individuals With Disabilities and Their Families

Date Enacted	Public Law No.	Name	Effects
1963	PL 88-164	Mental Retardation Facilities and Community Mental Health Centers Construction Act	Provided financial aid for building community-based facilities for persons with mental retardation and mental illness and authorized research centers and university-affiliated facilities (UAFs)
1963	PL 88-156	The Maternal and Child Health and Mental Retardation Planning Amendments	Established the Maternal and Child Health Program to improve prenatal care to high-risk women from low-income families
1970	PL 91-517	The Developmental Disabilities Services and Facilities Construction Amendments	Expands PL 88-164 into a comprehensive statute that also requires every state to establish a governor's council on developmental disabilities; first time the term "developmental disabilities" was used to replace "mental retardation"; persons with cerebral palsy and epilepsy are now eligible for services under this new definition
1972	PL 92-424	Economic Opportunity Act Amendments	Required Head Start enrollment to include a minimum of 10% of children with handicaps
1973	PL 93-112	Rehabilitation Act, Section 504	The first legislation to focus on rehabilitation services for people with severe disabilities; Section 504 established civil rights protection for all people with disabilities by prohibiting all recipients of federal funds from discrimination against individuals with disabilities
1978	PL 95-602	Rehabilitation Comprehensive Services and Developmental Disability Act	Defined developmental disabilities in functional terms and emphasized the severity and chronicity of these functional impairments; identified priority areas for state Developmental Disabilities Councils to address

(continued)

CHAPTER 6

TABLE 6-1. Federal Legislation Affecting Individuals With Disabilities and Their Families (continued)

Date Enacted	Public Law No.	Name	Effects
1984	PL 98-527	Developmental Disabilities Act Amendments	Amended the purpose of the Developmental Disability Act to ensure that individuals receive necessary services and to establish a coordination and monitoring system; definitions were added for independence, integration, supported employment, and employment-related activities
1987	PL 100-146	Developmental Disabilities Assistance & Bill of Rights Amendments	Revised priority service areas and added "family support service"; funds were pinpointed for training by university-affiliated programs to address the needs of persons with developmental disabilities in the area of early intervention
1988	PL 100-407	Technology Related Assistance for Individuals	Provided funds to assist states in developing technology-related assistance programs for individuals of all ages with disabilities; studies of financing issues and setting up a national information and referral network were also initiated
1990	PL 101-336	Americans with Disabilities Act	Extended Section 504 of the Rehabilitation Act of 1973; established protection for all persons with disabilities in the areas of employment, transportation, public services, public accommodations, and telecommunications regardless of how such services are funded (public or private)
1994	PL 103-218	Technology Related Assistance for Individuals Act Amendments	Stated that individuals with disabilities have a right to full inclusion and integration in the economic, political, social, cultural, and educational mainstream; provided funding to support systems change and advocacy activities to assist each state in developing and

(continued)

TABLE 6-1. Federal Legislation Affecting Individuals With Disabilities and Their Families (continued)

Date Enacted	Public Law No.	Name	Effects
			implementing a consumer-responsive, comprehensive statewide program of technology-related assistance for individuals of all ages who have disabilities
1994	PL 103-230	Developmental Disabilities Assistance & Bill of Rights Amendments	Defined assistive technology device, assistive technology service, community development activities, community living activities, community supports, culturally competent early intervention services, inclusion, and others
1996	PL 104-193	Personal Responsibility and Work Opportunity Reconciliation Act	Temporary Assistance to Needy Families (TANF) replaced Aid to Families with Dependent Children (AFDC); redefined childhood disability and eligibility for SSI; made provisions to assist families to enter into and retain employment; eliminated the guarantee of child care; granted flexibility to states

Early Intervention: Part C

Services to children birth through 2 years of age

Team establishes outcomes based on family concerns, needs, and priorities

Service plan is documented in the individualized family service plan (IFSP)

Physical therapy is a primary service provider; thus, a child can be eligible for physical therapy in isolation (Table 6-4)

Technology Related Assistance for Individuals With Disabilities Act (Tech Act)

Authorizes states to create a statewide system of technological assistance to children with disabilities

Carl D. Perkins Vocational and Applied Technology Education Act

Requires that children with disabilities be provided with vocational education in the LRE

As appropriate, vocational education is part of IEP

CHAPTER 6

TABLE 6-2. Federal Legislation Affecting Education Programs

Date Enacted	Public Law No.	Name	Effects
1975	PL 94-142	Education of the Handicapped Act	Provided the framework for special education for handicapped children ages 6 through 21; guaranteed free, appropriate public education; special education and related services; written individualized education programs (IEP); due process rights for parents; and placement in the least restrictive environment
1986	PL 99-457	Education of the Handicapped Act Amendments	Extended the above guarantees to 3- to 5-year-olds (Part B); established an early intervention discretionary program for infants and toddlers (0–3 years) and their families (Part C); stated design and implement services and supports with an emphasis on natural settings; mandated an individualized family services plan (IFSP) for all eligible children and their families
1991	PL 102-119	Individuals with Disabilities Education Act (IDEA)	Established a name change; used people-first language.
1997	PL 105-17	Individuals with Disabilities Education Act Amendments	Required states to establish performance goals and indicators for all children, including children with disabilities; children with disabilities must be included in state assessments of achievement; the IEP must explain the extent to which a child is not participating in regular education activities with children without disabilities; mediation must be made available to families; required states to monitor racial disproportionality in the identification and placement of children with disabilities; reinforced natural environments as service settings for early intervention

TABLE 6-3. Differences Between Early Intervention and School-Based Programs

Feature	Early Intervention	School
Program model	Family-centered	Child-centered
Primary program focus	Promotion/facilitation	Remedial/compensatory
Evaluation	Eligibility	Placement
	Current status	IEP development
Assessment	Programming needs	Not included
Family assessment	Voluntary to identify family strength, needs, and concerns related to infant	Not included
Services	Wide variety (medical, therapeutic, education, and psychosocial)	Instruction and related services necessary to benefit from special education
Review	Every 6 months	Annually
Location of services	Community-based	School-based
Agency responsibility	Variable	Education
Parent involvement	Integral team member	Passive participant
Planning document	IFSP	IEP

IEP, individualized education program; *IFSP,* individualized family services plan.

CIVIL RIGHTS

American with Disabilities Act (ADA)

Assures that individuals with disabilities are afforded equal access and reasonable accommodation in employment, education, and services in private and public sectors

Prohibits eligibility criteria that screen out or tend to screen out individuals with disabilities

Separate, special, or different programs designed to provide benefits to persons with disabilities cannot be used to restrict participation of persons with disabilities in general integrated activities

Rehabilitation Act Amendment of 1992

Ensures that individuals served are involved in the development of the individual written rehabilitation plan (IWRP)

Clarifies that vocational rehabilitation services include personnel assistance, transition, and supported employment

Section 504 applies to children with difficulties in learning that may not meet eligibility for special education services but require accommodations to benefit from the curriculum in the LRE

MEDICAL

Catastrophic Coverage Act

Allows states to obtain limited funds from Medicaid for services described in child's IEP or IFSP

TABLE 6-4. Comparison of Parts B and C of IDEA

Part B: Two groups of children are eligible to receive services under Part B:

- School age: 6- to 21-year-olds
  1) Having autism, deaf-blindness, deaf, hearing impairment, mental retardation, multiple disabilities, orthopedic impairments, other health impairments, visual impairment, serious emotional disturbance, specific learning disabilities, speech or language impairment, traumatic brain injury, and visual impairment including blindness and
  2) Who need special education and related services
- Preschool: 3- to 5-year-olds
  1) Having autism, deaf-blindness, deaf, hearing impairment, mental retardation, multiple disabilities, orthopedic impairments, other health impairments, visual impairment, serious emotional disturbance, specific learning disabilities, speech or language impairment, traumatic brain injury, and visual impairment including blindness and
  2) At state's discretion children showing developmental delays in physical, cognitive, communication, social/emotional, or adaptive development

Part C: Infants and toddlers who:

1) Show developmental delays (as defined by the State) in cognitive, physical, communication, social/emotional, or adaptive development
2) Have a diagnosed condition that has a high probability to result in developmental delay
3) At risk for developmental delay at state's discretion and
4) Who are in need of early intervention

Part B	Part C
Services	
Special education and related services documented on individualized education program (IEP) include but are not limited to	Early intervention services documented on individualized family service plans (IFSP) include but are not limited to
<ul><li>Assistive technology</li><li>Counseling services</li><li>Medical services (for diagnostic purposes)</li><li>Occupational therapy</li><li>Orientation and mobility</li><li>Parent counseling and training</li><li>Physical therapy</li><li>Psychology</li><li>Recreation</li><li>School health</li><li>Speech pathology</li><li>Transportation</li></ul>	<ul><li>Audiology</li><li>Service coordination</li><li>Family training and counseling</li><li>Health services</li><li>Medical services (for diagnostic purposes)</li><li>Nursing</li><li>Nutrition</li><li>Occupational therapy</li><li>Physical therapy</li><li>Psychology</li><li>Social work</li><li>Special instruction</li><li>Speech-language pathology</li><li>Early identification, screening, and assessment</li><li>Vision services</li><li>Assistive technology</li><li>Transportation</li></ul>

(continued)

TABLE 6-4. Comparison of Parts B and C of IDEA (continued)

Part B	Part C
Plans	

Part B	Part C
IEP	IFSP
• Child's present levels of educational performance	• Child's present levels of develop
• Annual goals, including short-term instructional objectives	• Family-directed assessment of the resources, priorities, and concerns of family
• Specific special education and related services to be provided to the child and the extent to which the child will be able to participate in regular education programs	• Major outcomes the child and family ar expected to achieve and the criteria, procedures, and timelines used to determine progress or need for modification
• Dates for initiation of services and the anticipated duration of the services	• Specific early intervention services necessary to meet the outcomes including:
• Appropriate objective criteria and evaluation procedures and schedules for determining, on at least an annual basis, whether the short-term instructional objectives are being achieved	— Frequency, intensity, location, and method of delivering services; payment arrangements, if any; other services not required by this act but needed by the child; and steps to secure these services from other sources
	• Projected dates for initiation of services and the anticipated duration of those services
	• Name of the service coordinator
	• Statement of the natural environments in which early intervention services shall be provided
Transition services	
• At age 16 every student will have an explicitly written plan for transition into employment or postsecondary education	• At local or state discretion, and with the concurrence of the family, 3- to 5-year-olds may have an IFSP or IEP, as long as IEP requirements are met
	• Steps to be taken to support the transition of the child at age 3 to preschool
Integration	
• Least restricted environment "to the maximum extent appropriate, children with disabilities . . . are educated with children who are not disabled, and that special classes, separate schooling, or other removal of children with disabilities from the regular educational environment occurs only when the nature or severity of the disability is such that education in regular classes with the use of supplementary aids and services cannot be achieved satisfactorily	• Natural environment "to the maximum extent appropriate, [services] are provided in natural environments, including the home and community settings . . . in which children without disabilities participate"

(continued)

CHAPTER 6

Comparison of Parts B and C of IDEA (continued)

Part B	Part C
Lead agency	
...tion agency	Governor-designated lead agency
Advisory panels	
Special Education Advisory Panel appointed by the governor	Interagency Coordinating Council
Members include	• Appointed by the governor
– Consumers	• At least 15 members but no more than 25 (unless approved)
– Parents	• Members include
– Teachers	– 20% parents
– Special education administrators	– 20% providers
– State and local officials	– 1 legislator
	– 1 personnel trainer
	– 1 state education agency representative
	– Representative of the 3- to 5-year-olds' program
	– 1 state insurance representative
	– Chair may be appointed by the governor from the members, or the governor shall have the members designate; no lead agency representative may serve as chair
	• Establishes a Federal Interagency Coordinating Council
Cost to parents	
No cost to parents (free, appropriate public education [FAPE])	State must establish a sliding fee scale if state law permits; however, families may not be denied services because of inability to pay; certain services must be provided at no cost: child find, evaluation and assessment, service coordination, development and review of IFSP, and procedural safeguards; if a state provides a FAPE from birth, all services are at no charge
With parental permission, Medicaid and other third-party insurance payers may be billed for medically related services, such as physical therapy	

Omnibus Budget Reconciliation Act (OBRA)

Expands early and periodic screening, diagnosis, and treatment (EPSDT)
Allows Medicaid funds to be used for medically necessary treatment

SERVICE DELIVERY

DRIVING FORCES OF SERVICE DELIVERY

System-centered: the strengths and needs of the system drive the delivery of services
Child-centered: the strengths and needs of the child drive the delivery of services
Family-centered: the strengths and needs of the family drive the delivery of services

SERVICE DELIVERY ENVIRONMENTS

A child with a disability or who is at risk for developing a disability due to environmental or biologic complications often receives physical therapy throughout many years and within many environments ⟩

Although treatment is individualized to meet the unique needs of each child and his or her family, the purpose of treatment and the design of a treatment plan are often dependent on the service delivery environment

Hospital

Neonatal Intensive Care Unit (NICU)

Provides developmental support to an infant

Primary treatment strategies include positioning programs, environmental adaptations, and incorporation of neuromotor activities into daily caregiving routines

Strong emphasis is placed on collaborating with nurses and medical staff members to minimize handling of the infant and physiologic stress

Pediatric Acute Care (Including Intensive Care)

Purposes are to decrease pain and discomfort, diminish effects on function from an acute illness or injury, and prepare child for hospital discharge

The traditional unidisciplinary, medical model of service delivery is common, although small multidisciplinary team models may be used

Discipline-specific treatment plans are common

Rehabilitation Center

Comprehensive and intensive treatment service using a multidisciplinary approach

Emphasis is on improving functional skills through exercise, activity, and assistive technology

Outpatient

Usually short-term services for children recovering from an acute illness or injury

For children with long-term disabilities, treatment as a hospital outpatient is often a transitional service while community-based services are secured

Early Intervention (EI)

Services are described under Part C of IDEA

For children from birth–2 years of age

May encompass services delivered in NICU, PICU, transitional care units

Services are family-centered and delivered in natural environments

Describes a system of care promoting inclusion of the child into naturally occurring activities and routines rather than a caregiving environment

Requires collaboration among service providers and interagency cooperation
* Prevent duplication of services
* Promote consistency among care providers

Physical therapy is a primary service provider
* Can be a single service

IFSP
* Outcome-based care plans
* Specific therapeutic goals and objectives derived from outcomes using a top-down assessment strategy (see Fig. 3-1)

CHAPTER 6

Education
Special Education
Educationally based services designed for children with a disability that affects their educational achievement, performance, or participation in the curriculum in the LRE

Services are described under Part B of IDEA

Physical therapy is considered a related service

- Service designed and delivered in a manner that enables a child to benefit from special education within the LRE
- Therapeutic plans must support the implementation of with IEP
- Integrated service delivery system within naturally occurring school-based activities and routines
- Therapists cooperate, collaborate, and consult with a variety of educational service personnel

Private Practice
The pediatric private practitioner often serves children and families in a variety of settings in addition to outpatient facilities

Therapists assume responsibility to provide service under the legislative and regulatory constraints of the service delivery environment

Generally provide services under two types of contractual agreements: directly with a child's family or with a service provider organization (local educational agency, hospital, early intervention program) (Table 6-5)

TEAM COMPOSITION
Team-based service delivery is advocated to meet the diverse needs of the child

Teams consist of two or more individuals who provide intervention (Table 6-6)

MODELS OF SERVICE DELIVERY
Focus of Service Delivery
Prevention
Intervention planned to prevent the effects of biologic or environmental factors on development

Promotion
Intervention designed to promote the acquisition of motor skills, activities of daily living, or other relevant skills

Providers create an environment that promotes skill development to emerge within naturally occurring activities

Remediation
Intervention to improve components of movement and to facilitate the acquisition of developmental milestones or other motor activities lost to injury, illness, or biologic insult

Strategies are designed to alleviate identified problems, impairments, and functional limitations

Compensation
Minimizes the effects of a disability through the use of external devices or assistive technology or instruction in compensatory skills to promote function

TABLE 6-5. Factors That May Influence the Status of an Employee or Independent Contractor

Employee	Contractor
Assuming no employment contract, discharge of or resignation by an individual before completion of work would not be breach of contract	Discharge of or resignation by individual before completion of work would be breach of contract
Employer furnishes the tools, materials, or equipment to perform the work	Individual furnishes his or her own tools, materials, or equipment
Services are performed on employer's premises or where instructed by employer	Unless agreed upon, individual is not required to work on employer's premise
Individual receives fixed wage	Individual receives a sum payment for work; has a possibility of sustaining a loss
Individual has continuing relationship with employer	Individual is permitted to employ assistants, with exclusive right to supervise and delegate to them
	Individual is hired to do specific job or piece of work
Contract is for purchase of labor	Contract is for purchase of product
Employer provides opportunities for individual to receive periodic or sporadic training, formally or informally	Contractor responsible to participate in training on an ongoing basis
Relationship exists between services of individual and function and scope of employer's business; success of business may depend on actions of individual	Services performed by individual are not in the usual course of employer's business
Hours of work are established by employer	Individual determines when work will be done
Individual is required to submit regular oral or written reports to employer	Individual is not required to account for his or her time

Emphasis is on designing a strategy to promote task performance or participation in an activity

Method
Isolated
Treatment of therapist-identified deficits and needs outside the child's natural environment (clinic, separate classroom, separate area within class)

Focus is usually remedial

Integrated
Services provided during naturally occurring activities and routines

Consistent with the LRE mandate of IDEA

Requires collaboration among team members

3LE 6-6. Service Provision Teams

	Multidisciplinary	Interdisciplinary	Trandisciplinary
;uiding philosophy	Team members recognize the importance of contributions from other disciplines	Team members are willing and able to develop, share, and be responsible for providing services that are a part of the total service plan	Team members make a commitment to teach, learn, and work together across discipline boundaries to implement unified service plan
Examination, evaluation, assessment	Completed separately by team members	Completed separately by team members	Team members and family conduct a comprehensive developmental assessment together
Parent participation	Parents meet with individual team members	Parents meet with team or team representative	Parents are full, active, and participating members of the team
Service plan development	Team members develop separate plans for their disciplines	Team members share their separate plans with one another	Team members, including parents, develop a service plan based on family priorities, needs, and resources
Service plan implementation	Team members implement the part of the service plan related to their discipline	Team members implement their section of the plan and incorporate other sections when possible	A primary service provider is assigned to implement the plan with the family
Service plan responsibility	Team members are responsible for implementing their sections of the plan	Team members are responsible for sharing information with one another and for implementing their section of the plan	Team members are responsible and accountable for how the primary service provider implements the plan
Lines of communication	Informal lines	Periodic case-specific team meetings	Regular team meetings during which information, knowledge, and skills are shared among team members
Staff development	Independent and within their disciplines	Independent within and outside their disciplines	An integral component is for learning across disciplines and team building

Adapted with permission from Woodruff, G., & McGonigal, M. J. (1990). Early intervention team approaches: The transdisciplinary model. In J. Jordan, J. Gallegher, P. Hutinger, & M. Karnes (Eds.), *Early Childhood Special Education: Birth to Three* (p.196). Baltimore, MD: Paul H. Brookes.

Direct

Hands-on treatment strategies designed by therapists which can be delivered safely by therapist only

Typical for the isolated service delivery model but can also be a component of integrated model to

- Assess a child
- Determine intervention strategies
- Train others
- Solve problems
- Modify program

Consultation

Therapists provides information and expertise to assist the team in solving a specific problem

Services may be infrequent and of short duration or as time-consuming as direct services

Used to modify/adapt materials or positions

Therapist is responsible for ensuring that accepted suggestions are carried out appropriately by appropriate personnel

Collaborative-consultation is preferred method of consultation

Monitoring

Therapist instructs/supervises others in an intervention plan and provides ongoing support and guidance to the implementers to ensure successful implementation

Promotes embedding therapeutic strategies into naturally occurring activities and routines

Provides opportunities for generalization

Promotes ongoing team interaction and problem-solving

■ DOCUMENTATION

PURPOSE

Facilitates efficacious treatment

Method of communication among providers of service, families, and payers of service

Justifies reimbursement

Legal record

Promotes accountability

CONSIDERATIONS

The following may influence the type and frequency of documentation required

- Service delivery setting
- Needs of individual children
- Payers of service
- Team model
- Government regulations
- Professional licensing regulations

RUMBA

Developed by the Quality Assurance Division of American Occupational Therapy Association (AOTA)

- Is documentation *r*elevant?
- Is documentation *u*nderstandable?

documentation stated in *measurable* terms?
Does documentation contain *behavioral* data?
Are plans *achievable*?

DOCUMENTATION PLANS

Hospital/Rehabilitation Centers
Problem-Orientated Medical Record (POMR)

SOAP
- Subjective
- Objective
- Assessment
- Plan

Non-SOAP
- Problem
- Plan
- Results

Early Intervention
IFSP

Team-developed intervention plan

Family-centered
- Family members are equal members of decision-making team
- Needs and concerns of the family drive plan development

Special Education
IEP (Table 6-7)

Team-developed intervention plan

Family is a participant in the team process

Outcomes are specific to the needs of the child

Community-Based Post-Educational Programs
Individualized Habilitation Plans (IHP)

Similar to IFSP, IEP

Primarily developed for adults with developmental disabilities who have graduated from
educational programs

Focus is on vocational programming, independent living, functional skill training, and activities of daily living

Behavioral Objectives

Statements of what behavior is expected of the child receiving therapy

Five components
- The child or recipient of therapy is identified
- The target or expected behavior is determined
- The conditions under which the behavior will be measured are stated
- Criteria determining success are stated
- The time frame for achieving the outcome is listed

Usually individualized to meet the unique needs of the child, family, and service delivery
system

TABLE 6-7. Comparison of the IEP and IFSP

Component	IEP	IFSP
Performance	Present level of educational performance	Present level of development
Family	Family's needs are not part of the IEP	With agreement from family, includes a statement of the family's strengths and needs related to enhancing the development of the child
Goals	Annual goals Short-term objectives	Annual outcomes
Services	Education and related services	Early intervention
Setting	Least restrictive education environment; inclusion	Natural settings
Medical services	No provision	Statement of medical services necessary to meet child's needs
Timelines	Projected dates for initiation of services and the anticipated duration of services	Projected dates for initiation of services and the anticipated duration of services
Documentation	Objective criteria, evaluation procedures, and schedules for determining whether objectives are being met annually	Criteria, procedures, and timelines on semiannual basis
Service coordinator	No provision	Service coordinator indicated
Transition of planning	Documents activities that promote movement from school to postsecondary activities beginning at age 14	Steps are outlined that will support the child, family, and team in moving from early intervention to preschool

IEP, individualized education program; *IFSP,* individualized family services plan.

Goal Attainment Scaling (GAS)

Requires that goals be written in measurable, observable terms, with specifications of the conditions in which the objective will be judged as met and the time frame in which the objective will be completed

Includes not only the expected outcome but also two outcomes that do not meet criteria and two that go beyond the minimal criteria or expected attainment

System available to determine standard scores

CODING SYSTEMS

Standardized notations indicating the diagnosis of the client and the procedures or services provided

Because coding systems change on a regular basis, therapists must keep abreast of these modifications, which include additions and deletions

CHAPTER 6

TABLE 6-8. Commonly Used ICD-9 Codes for Children With Disabilities

Name	Number	Name	Number
Abnormal movement	781.0	Hypertonia	
Anomalies of skull and face hair	756.0	Fetus/newborn	779.8
Ataxia	781.3	Hypotonia	358.8
Brachial plexus	353.0	Congenital	779.8
Fetus/newborn	767.6	Infantile muscular	359.0
Klumpke	767.6	Muscle	728.9
Cerebral palsy		Laryngospasm	478.75
Noncongenital noninfantile	344.8	Legg-Perthes	732.1
Due to vascular lesion	438	Microcephalus	742.1
Congenital, infantile, spastic	343.9	Monoplegic	343.3
Athetoid	333.7	Motor apraxia	784.69
Diplegia	343.0	Muscular dystrophy	359
Hemiplegia	343.1	Duchenne	359.1
Congenital hip dislocation		Hereditary progressive	359.1
Unilateral	754.3	Congenital	359.0
Bilateral	754.31	Myotonic	359.2
Dandy-Walker cyst	742.3	Limb-girdle	359.1
With spina bifida	741.0	Muscle weakness	728.9
Dentofacial anomaly	524.0–	Neurologic neglect	781.8
	524.9	Pes varus, congenital	754.5
Developmental delay	783.4	Spina bifida	741
Developmental learning delays	315–	Aperta	741.9
	315.9	Unspecified region	741.0
Delayed motor coordination	315.4	Cervical	741.1
Difficulty walking	719.7	Dorsal	741.2
Down syndrome	758.0	Lumbar	741.3
Dyspraxia	781.3	Torticollis	
Equinovarus, congenital	754.51	Spastic	723.5
Facial palsy	351.0	Congenital	754.1
Newborn	767.5	Sternocleidomastoid	754.1
Glossopharyngeal	352.2	Due to birth injury	767.8
Gait abnormality	781.2	Spinal muscular atrophy	
Hydrocephalus	742.1	Werdnig-Hoffman	335.0

This list is not exhaustive. It contains some of the most commonly used codes. The reader should see the ICD-9 code book for further information.

International Classification of Diseases, Ninth Revision, Clinical Modification (ICD-9-CM) (Table 6-8)

Classifies illness, injuries, and services

Provider lists as specifically as possible the principal and secondary diagnoses

The diagnostic description of the current problem should be defined by

- Client's subjective problem/complaint
- Date of onset of problem

- Objective examination of client confirming diagnosis
- Functional outcomes

V codes: identify visits with practitioners for factors influencing health s
fitting for an orthosis or a walker, but not treatment of an acute disease

Current Procedural Terminology (CPT)

Can be found in

- *Health Care Financing Administration's Common Procedure Coding System* (H
  Level II)
- *Diagnostic and Statistical Manual of Mental Disorders, 4th Edition* (DSM-IV)

Resources

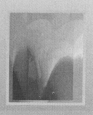

GOVERNMENT AGENCIES

Administration on Developmental Disabilities
Administration for Children and Families
U.S. Department of Health and Human Services
Mail Stop: HHH 300-F
370 L'Enfant Promenade, SW
Washington, DC 20447
phone: 202-690-6590
http://www.acf.dhhs.gov/programs/add/

Agency for Health Care Research and Quality
2101 E. Jefferson Street, Suite 501
Rockville, MD 20852
phone: 301-594-1364
www.ahcpr.gov

Communication and Information Services
(Formerly Clearinghouse on Disability Information)
Office of Special Education and Rehabilitative Services
Room 3132, Switzer Building
330 C Street, SW
Washington, DC 20202-2524
phone: 202-205-8241

Department of Health and Human Services
200 Independence Avenue, SW
Washington, DC 20201
phone: 877-696-6779
www.os.dhhs.gov
www.healthfinder.gov
Division of Services for Children with Special Health Needs
www.mchb.hrsa.gov/html/dscshn.html

Head Start Bureau
Administration on Children, Youth and Families
U.S. Department of Health & Human Services
PO Box 1182
Washington, DC 20013
phone: 202-645-3060
www.acf.dhhs.gov/programs/hsb/

National Arthritis and Musculoskeletal and Skin Diseases Information Clearinghouse
1 AMS Circle
Bethesda, MD 20892-3675
phone: 301-495-4484
TTY: 301-565-2966
www.nih.gov/niams

Office of Special Education and Rehabilitative Services (OSERS)
330 C Street, SW
Mary E. Switzer Building
Washington, DC 20202
phone: 202-205-5507
www.ed.gov/offices/OSERS/

President's Committee on Employment of People with Disabilities
1331 F Street, NW
Washington, DC 20004
phone: 202-376-6200
TDD: 202-376-6205
fax: 202-376-6219

President's Committee on Mental Retardation
370 L'Enfant Promenade, SW, Suite 701
Washington, DC 20447
phone: 202-619-0634
fax: 202-205-9519
www.acf.dhhs.gov/programs/pcmr/

U.S. Architectural and Transportation Barriers Compliance Board
1331 F Street, NW, Suite 1000
Washington, DC 20004
phone: 202-272-5434, 800-872-2253
fax: 202-272-5447

PROFESSIONAL ORGANIZATIONS

American Academy for Cerebral Palsy and Developmental Medicine
6300 North River Road, Suite 727
Rosemont, IL 60018-4226
phone: 847-698-1635
fax: 847-823-0536
www.aacpdm.org/

American Academy of
Pediatric Dentistry
211 East Chicago Avenue,
   #700
Chicago, IL 60611-2663
phone: 312-337-2169
fax: 312-337-6329
www.aapd.org/

American Academy of
Pediatrics
141 Northwest Point
   Boulevard
Elk Grove Village, IL
   60007-1098
phone: 847-434-4000
fax: 847-434-8000
www.aap.org

American Association on
Mental Retardation
(AAMR)
444 N. Capitol Street, NW,
   Suite 846
Washington, DC 20001
phone: 202-387-1968
fax: 202-387-2193

American Occupational
Therapy Association
4720 Montgomery Lane
PO Box 31220
Bethesda, MD 20824-1220
phone: 301-652-2682
TTD: 800-377-8555
fax: 301-652-7711
www.aota.org/

American Physical
Therapy Association
1111 North Fairfax Street
Alexandria, VA 22314-1488
phone: 703-684-2782
TTD: 703-683-6748
fax: 703-684-7343
www.apta.org/

American Speech-Language-
Hearing Association
10801 Rockville Pike
Rockville, MD 20852
phone: 301-897-5700,
   800-498-2071
TTY: 301-897-5700
fax: 301-571-0457
www.asha.org/

American Therapeutic
Recreation Association
PO Box 15215
Hattiesburg, MS 39404-5215
phone: 800-553-0304
www.atra-tr.org

Association for Persons with
Severe Handicaps (TASH)
29 W. Susquehanna Avenue,
   Suite 210
Baltimore, MD 21204
phone: 410-828-8274
fax: 410-828-6706
www.tash.org

Association of Birth Defects
in Children
827 Irma Street
Orlando, FL 32803
phone: 407-629-1466,
   800-313-2232
fax: 407-629-1466

Association on Higher
Education and Disability
PO Box 21192
Columbus, OH 43221
phone: 614-488-4972
TTY: 614-488-4972
fax: 614-488-1174

Commission on Mental and
Physical Disability Law
740 15th Street, NW
Washington, DC 20005
phone: 202-662-1570
TTY: 202-662-1012
fax: 202-662-1032
www.abanet.org/disability/h
ome.html

International Association for
Disability and Oral Health
(Formerly the International
   Association of Dentistry
   for the Handicapped)
The Ohio State University
   College of Dentistry
305 West 12th Avenue
Columbus, OH 43218
phone: 614-292-1232
fax: 614-292-4522
www.iadh.org/

Neuro-Developmental
Treatment Association
1550 South Coast Highway,
   Suite 201
Laguna Beach, CA 92651
phone: 800-869-9295
fax: 949-376-3456
www.ndta.org/index.html

PAM Assistance Center
1023 S. US Route 27
St. Johns, MI 48879
phone: 800-274-7426
fax: 517-224-0957

Sensory Integration
International
1514 Cabrillo Avenue
Torrance, CA 90501
phone: 310-320-2335
fax: 310-320-9982
www.home.earthlink.net/
   ~sensoryint/

ADVOCACY AND EDUCATION

ACCENT on Information
PO Box 700
Bloomington, IL 61702
phone: 309-378-2961
fax: 309-378-4420

Access Board
1331 F Street, NW, Suite
1000
Washington, DC 20004-
1111
phone: 202-272-5434,
800-872-2253
TTY: 202-272-5449,
800-993-2822
fax: 202-272-5447
www.access-board.gov

Alexander Graham Bell
Association for the Deaf
3417 Volta Place NW
Washington, DC 20007
phone: 202-337-5220
(Voice/TTY)
www.agbell.org

American Bar Association
Center on Children and the
Law
740 15th Street, NW
9th Floor
Washington, DC 20061
phone: 202-662-1720
fax: 202-662-1032

American Civil Liberties
Union Children's Rights
Project
132 W. 43rd Street
New York, NY 10036
phone: 212-944-9800
fax: 212-921-7916

American Council on Rural
Special Education (ACRES)
Kansas State University
2323 Anderson Avenue,
Suite 226
Manhattan, KS 66502
phone: 785-532-2737
www.ksu.edu/acres

Americans with Disabilities
Act Information Line
U.S. Department of Justice
Civil Rights Division
PO Box 66118
Washington, DC 20035-
6118
phone: 202-514-0301,
800-514-0301
TDD: 800-514-0383
www.usdoj.gov/crt/ada/
adahom1.htm

The Arc
(Formerly, Association for
Retarded Citizens of the
U.S.)
1730 K Street, NW, Suite
1212
Washington, DC 20006
phone: 202-785-3388
fax: 202-467-4179
www.thearc.org/welcome.
html

Center for Universal Design
NC State University
School of Design
Box 8613
219 Oberlin Road (delivery
address)
Raleigh, NC 27695-8613
phone: 919-515-3082
TTY: 919-515-3082
fax: 919-515-3023
www2.ncsu.edu/ncsu/design/
cud

Children's Defense Fund
25 E. Street, NW
Washington, DC 20001
phone: 202-628-8787,
800-233-1200
fax: 202-662-3510
www.tmm.com/cdf/index.
html

Council for Exceptional
Children (CEC)
1920 Association Drive
Reston, VA 20191-1589
phone: 703-620-3660,
888-232-7733
fax: 703-264-9494
TTY: 703-264-9446
www.cec.sped.org/index.
htm

Disability Rights and
Education Defense Fund
2212 Sixth Street
Berkeley, CA 94710
phone: 510-644-2555
(Voice/TTY)
fax: 510-841-8645
www.dredf.org

Institute for Children,
Youth, and Families (ISIS)
27 Kellogg Center
Michigan State University
East Lansing, MI 48824-
1022
phone: 517-353-6617
fax: 517-355-4565
www.isisweb.org

International Society on
Early Intervention (ISEI)
www.depts.washington.edu/
isei

Kids on the Block
9385 C Gerwig Lane
Columbia, MD 21046
phone: 800-368-5437
fax: 410-290-9358
www.kotb.com

Learning Disabilities
Association of America
(LDA)
4156 Library Road
Pittsburgh, PA 15234
phone: 412-341-1515
fax: 412-344-0224
www.ldanatl.org

National Association of
Developmental Disabilities
Councils
1234 Massachusetts Avenue,
NW, Suite 103
Washington, DC 20005
phone: 202-347-1234
fax: 202-347-4023
www.igc.org/NADDC/

National Association of
Private Schools for
Exceptional Children
(NAPSEC)
1522 K Street, NW, Suite
1032
Washington, DC 20005
phone: 202-408-3338
www.napsec.com

National Association of
Protection and Advocacy
Systems (NAPAS)
900 Second Street, NE, Suite
211
Washington, DC 20002
phone: 202-408-9514
TTY: 202-408-9521
www.protectionandadvocacy.
com/

National Association of
the Deaf
814 Thayer Avenue
Silver Spring, MD 20910-
4500
phone: 301-587-1788
TTY: 301-587-1789
fax: 301-587-1791
www.nad.org/

National Center on
Accessibility
Indiana University
2805 East 10th Street, Suite
190
Bloomington, IN 47408-
2698
phone: 812-856-4422
TTY: 812-856-4421
fax: 812-856-4480
www.ncaonline.org

Parent Education and
Advocacy Training Center
10340 Democracy Lane
Fairfax, VA 22030
phone: 703-691-7826
fax: 703-691-8148

Pathways Awareness
Foundation
123 North Wacker Drive
Chicago, IL 60606
phone: 800-955-2445
TTY: 312-236-7411
www.pathwaysawareness.org

Technical Assistance
Alliance for Parent Centers
(the Alliance)
PACER Center
4826 Chicago Avenue South
Minneapolis, MN 55417-
1098
phone: 612-827-2966,
888-248-0822
TTY: 612-827-7770
www.taalliance.org

PARENT SUPPORT GROUPS

Alliance of Genetic Support
Groups
4301 Connecticut, NW,
Suite 404
Washington, DC 20008
phone: 202-966-5557,
800-336-4363 (helpline
only)
fax: 202-966-8553
www.geneticalliance.org

American Society for Deaf
Children
PO Box 3355
Gettysburg, PA 17325
phone: 717-334-7922
(Voice/TTY) ,
800-942-2732
www.deafchildren.org

Association for Children
with Down Syndrome, Inc
(ACDS)
4 Fern Place
Plainview, NY 11803
phone: 516-933-4700
fax: 516-933-9524
www.acds.org

Compassionate Friends
PO Box 3696
Oak Brook, IL 60522
phone: 630-990-0010
fax: 630-990-0246
pages.prodigy.com/CA/
lycq97a/1ycq97tcf.html

Exceptional Parent
PO Box 3000
Department EP
Denville, NJ 07834
phone: 800-247-8080

Hydrocephalus Support
Group
PO Box 4236
Chesterfield, MO 63006
phone: 314-532-8228
fax: 314-995-4108

Life Services for the
Handicapped
352 Park Avenue, Suite 703
New York, NY 10010
phone: 212-532-6740,
800-995-0066
www.disabledandalone.org

Mothers United for Moral
Support, Inc.
150 Cluster Street
Green Bay, WI 54301
phone: 414-336-5333

National Association
for Parents of the
Visually Impaired
PO Box 317
Watertown, MA 02272
phone: 800-562-6265

National Parent to Parent
Support and Information
System, Inc.
PO Box 907
Blue Ridge, GA 30513
phone: 706-374-3822,
    800-651-1151
www.nppsis.org

Parents Helping Parents:
The Parent-Directed Family
Resource Center for
Children with Special Needs
3041 Olcott Street
Santa Clara, CA 95054
phone: 408-727-5775
www.php.com

DISABILITY-SPECIFIC
ORGANIZATIONS

National Adrenal Diseases
Foundation
505 Northern Boulevard
Great Neck, NY 11021
phone: 516-487-4992
medhlp.netuse.net/www/
    nadf.htm

CDC National AIDS Hotline
American Society Health
    Association
PO Box 13827
Research Triangle Park, NC
    27709
phone: 800-342-2437
TTY: 800-243-7889
fax: 919-361-4855
www.ashastd.org

National Pediatric & Family
HIV Resource Center
30 Bergen Street, ADMC-4
Newark, NJ 07107
phone: 973-972-0410,
    800-362-0071
fax: 973-972-0399
www.wdcnet.com/pedsaids

American Amputee
Foundation
PO Box 250218
Little Rock, AR 72225
phone: 501-666-2523
fax: 501-666-8367

Amputee Coalition of
America
900 E. Hill Avenue, Suite
    285
Knoxville, TN 37915
phone: 423-524-8772,
    888-267-5669
www.amputee-coalition.org

National Amputation
Foundation
38–40 Church Street
Malvem, NY 11565
phone: 516-887-3600
fax: 516-887-3667

Angelman Syndrome
Foundation
PO Box 12437
Gainesville, FL 32604
phone: 800-432-6435
www.angelman.org

American Anorexia Bulimia
Association
165 West 46 Street, #1108
New York, NY 10036
phone: 212-575-6200
www.members.aol.com/
    amanbu

Anorexia Nervosa and
Related Eating Disorders, Inc.
PO Box 5102
Eugene, OR 97405
phone: 800-931-2237
www.anred.com

Anxiety Disorders
Association of America
11900 Parklawn Drive,
    #100
Rockville, MD 20852-2624
phone: 301-231-9350
fax: 301-231-7392
www.adaa.org

Aplastic Anemia Foundation
of America, Inc.
PO Box 613
Annapolis, MD 21404-0613
phone: 410-867-0242,
    800-747-2820
fax: 410-867-0240
www.aplastic.org

American Juvenile Arthritis
Organization
1330 W. Peachtree Street
Atlanta, GA 30309
phone: 404-872-7100,
    800-283-7800
fax: 404-872-9559

Asthma and Allergy
Foundation of America
1233 20th Street, NW, Suite
    402
Washington, DC 20036
phone: 800-727-8462
fax: 202-466-8940
www.aafa.org/

National Ataxia Foundation
2600 Fernbrook Lane, Suite
    119
Minneapolis, MN 55447
phone: 763-553-0020
fax: 763-553-0167
www.ataxia.org

The ADHD Challenge
PO Box 488
West Peabody, MA 01985
phone: 800-233-2322

Children and Adults with
Attention-Deficit/
Hyperactivity Disorder
(CHADD)
8181 Professional Place,
Suite 201
Landover, MD 20785
phone: 301-306-7070,
800-233-4050
fax: 301-306-7090
www.chadd.org

National Attention Deficit
Disorder Association
1788 Second Street, Suite
200
Highland Park, IL 60035
phone: 847-432-2332
fax: 847-432-5874
www.add.org

Autism Research Institute
4182 Adams Avenue
San Diego, CA 92116
phone: 619-281-7165
fax: 619-563-6840
www.autism.com/autism

Autism Society of America
7910 Woodmont Avenue,
Suite 300
Bethesda, MD 20814-3015
phone: 301-657-0881,
800-3AUTISM
fax: 301-657-0869
www.autism-society.org/

National Autism Hotline/
Autism Services Center
605 9th Street, Prichard
Building
PO Box 507
Huntington, WV 25710
phone: 304-525-8014
fax: 304-525-8026

American Autoimmune
Related Diseases Association
Michigan National Bank
Building
15475 Gratiot Avenue
Detroit, MI 48205
phone: 313-371-8600,
800-598-4668
www.aarda.org

Bell's Palsy Research
Foundation
9121 E. Tanque Verde, Suite
105–286
Tucson, AZ 85749
phone: 520-749-4614

American Council of the
Blind
1155 15th Street, NW, Suite
720
Washington, DC 20005
phone: 202-467-5081,
800-424-8666
fax: 202-467-5085
www.acb.org

American Foundation for
the Blind (AFB)
11 Penn Plaza, Suite 300
New York, NY 10001
phone: 800-232-5463
TTY: 212-502-7662
www.afb.org

Keystone Blind Association
1230 Stambaugh Avenue
Sharon, PA 16146
phone: 724-347-5501
fax: 724-347-2204
www.keystoneblind.org

National Association for
Visually Handicapped
3201 Balboa Street
San Francisco, CA 94121
phone: 415-221-3201
fax: 415-221-8754
www.navh.org
or
22 West 21st Street
New York, NY 10010
phone: 212-889-3141
fax: 212-727-2931

National Braille Press
88 St. Stephen Street
Boston, MA 02115
phone: 617-266-6160,
888-965-8965
fax: 617-437-0456
www.nbp.org

National Federation for
the Blind
1800 Johnson Street
Baltimore, MD 21230
phone: 410-659-9314
www.nfb.org

National Library Services
for the Blind & Physically
Handicapped
The Library of Congress
1291 Taylor Street, NW
Washington, DC 20542
phone: 202-707-5100
TDD: 202-707-0744
fax: 202-707-0712
e-mail: nls@loc.gov
www.loc.gov/nls

Recording for the Blind
and Dyslexic
20 Roszel Road
Princeton, NJ 08540
phone: 609-452-0606,
800-221-4792
fax: 609-520-7990
www.rfbd.org

American Association of the
Deaf-Blind
814 Thayer Avenue, Suite
302
Silver Spring, MD 20910-
4500
phone: 800-735-2258
TTY: 301-588-6545
fax: 301-588-8705
www.tr.wosc.osshe.edu/
dblink/aadb.htm

National Family Association
for Deaf-Blind
111 Middle Neck Road
Sands Point, NY 11050
phone: 800-255-0411, ext.
275
TTY: 516-944-8637
fax: 516-944-7302

American Society for
Deaf Children
PO Box 3355
Gettysburg, PA 17325
phone: 717-334-7922
(voice/TTY),
800-942-2732 (parent
hotline)
fax: 717-334-8808
www.deafchildren.org

Captioned Films/Videos
5000 Park Street, N
St. Petersburg, FL 33709
phone: 800-237-6213
TTY: 800-237-6213
fax: 813-541-7571

John Tracy Clinic for
Preschool Deaf Children
806 W. Adams Boulevard
Los Angeles, CA 90007
phone: 213-747-2924,
800-522-4582
(voice/TTY)
www.jogntracyclinic.org

National Association of
the Deaf
814 Thayer Avenue
Silver Spring, MD 20910
phone: 301-587-1788
TTY: 301-587-1789
fax: 301-587-1791
www.nad.com

BMT Newsletter (Bone
Marrow Transplant)
1985 Spruce Avenue
Highland Park, IL 60035
phone: 847-831-1913
www.bmtnews.org

Brain Injury Association
(Formerly the National
Head Injury Foundation)
105 North Alfred Street
Alexandria, VA 22314
phone: 703-236-6000,
800-444-6443
fax: 703-236-6001
www.biausa.org

American Brain Tumor
Association
2720 River Road
Des Plaines, IL 60018
phone: 847-827-9910,
800-886-2282 (Patient
Services)
fax: 847-827-9918
www.abta.org/

Brain Tumor Foundation
for Children
2231 Perimeter Park Drive,
Suite 9
Atlanta, GA 30341
phone: 770-458-5554
fax: 770-458-5467

Children's Brain Diseases
Foundation
350 Parnassus Avenue, Suite
900
San Francisco, CA 94117
phone: 415-565-6259
fax: 415-863-3452

Children's Brain Tumor
Foundation
274 Madison Avenue, Suite
1301
New York, NY 10016
phone: 212-448-9491
fax: 212-448-1022
www.peds-neuro-web.med.
nyu.edu/cbbtf/cbtf_hp.
htm

National Brain Tumor
Foundation
414 Thirteenth Street, Suite
700
Oakland, CA 94612
phone: 510-839-9777,
800-934-2873
fax: 510-839-9779
www.braintumor.org

Phoenix Society for
Burn Survivors
33 Main Street, Suite 403
Nashua, NH 03060
phone: 603-889-3000,
800-888-2876
fax: 603-889-4688
www.burns-phoenix-
society.org

American Cancer Society
1599 Clifton Road, NE
Atlanta, GA 30329
phone: 404-320-3333,
800-277-2345
www.cancer.org

Cancer Net
NCI Public Inquiries Office
Building 31, Room 10A03
31 Center Drive, MSC 2580
Bethesda, MD 20892-2580
phone: 800-422-6237
TTY: 800-332-8615
fax: 800-624-2511
www.cancernet.nci.nih.gov

Candlelighters Childhood
Cancer Foundation
7910 Woodmont Avenue,
Suite 460
Bethesda, MD 20814
phone: 301-657-8400,
800-366-2223
fax: 301-718-2686

American Academy for
Cerebral Palsy and
Developmental Medicine
6300 North River Road,
Suite 727
Rosemont, IL 60018
phone: 708-698-1635
fax: 708-823-0536

United Cerebral Palsy
Association
1660 L Street, NW, Suite
700
Washington, DC 20036-
5602
phone: 202-776-0406,
800-USA-5-UCP
TTY: 202-973-7197
fax: 202-776-0414
www.ucpa.org

Charcot-Marie-Tooth
Association
601 Upland Avenue
Upland, PA 19015
phone: 610-499-7486,
800-606-2682
fax: 610-499-7487
www.charcot-marie-tooth.
org

Chronic Fatigue and
Immune Dysfunction
Syndrome Association
PO Box 220398
Charlotte, NC 28222-0398
phone: 704-365-2343,
800-442-3437
fax: 704-365-9755
www.cfids.org

AboutFace USA
PO Box 93
Limekiln, PA 19535
phone: 800-225-3223
fax: 610-689-4479

Cleft Palate Foundation
104 South Estes Drive, Suite
204
Chapel Hill, NC 27514
phone: 919-933-9044,
800-242-5338
fax: 919-933-9604
www.cleftline.org

Craniofacial Foundation of
America
975 East Third Street
Chattanooga, TN 37403
phone: 423-778-919,
800-418-3223
fax: 423-778-8172
www.erlanger.org/cranio

Children's Craniofacial
Association
PO Box 280297
Dallas, TX 75243-4522
phone: 972-994-9902,
800-535-3643
www.masterlink.com/
children/

FACES: The National
Craniofacial Association
PO Box 11082
Chattanooga, TN 37401
phone: 423-266-1632,
800-332-2372
www.faces-cranio.org

Pediatric Crohn's & Colitis
Association
PO Box 188
Newton, MA 02168
phone/fax: 617-489-5854

Cystic Fibrosis Foundation
6931 Arlington Road
Bethesda, MD 20814
phone: 301-951-4422,
800-344-4823
www.cff.org

American Diabetes
Association
1701 N. Beauregard Street
Alexandria, VA 22311
phone: 703-549-1500,
800-342-2383
www.diabetes.org

Association for Children
with Down Syndrome
2616 Martin Avenue
Bellmore, NY 11710
phone: 516-221-4700
fax: 516-221-5867

National Association for
Down's Syndrome
PO Box 4542
Oak Brook, IL 60522
phone: 630-325-9112
www.nads.org

National Down Syndrome
Congress
7000 Peachtree-Dunwoody
Road, NE
Lake Ridge 400 Office Park,
Building #5, Suite 100
Atlanta, GA 30328
phone: 770-604-9500,
800-232-6372
www.ndsccenter.org

National Down Syndrome
Society
666 Broadway, 8th Floor
New York, NY 10012-2317
phone: 212-460-9330,
800-221-4602
fax: 212-979-2837
www.ndss.org

Dyslexia Research
Institute, Inc.
4745 Centerville Road
Tallahassee, FL 32308
phone: 904-893-2216
fax: 904-893-2440

International Dyslexia
Association
(Formerly the Orton
  Dyslexia Society)
Chester Building #382
8600 LaSalle Road
Baltimore, MD 21286-2044
phone: 410-296-0232,
  800-222-3123
www.interdys.org

Dystonia Medical Research
Foundation
One E Wacker Drive, Suite
  2430
Chicago, IL 60601
phone: 312-755-0198
fax: 312-803-0138
www.dystonia-foundation.
  org

American Epilepsy Society
638 Prospect Avenue
Hartford, CT 06105-4240
phone: 860-586-7505
fax: 860-586-7550
www.aesnet.org

Epilepsy Foundation of
America
4351 Garden City Drive, 5th
  Floor
Landover, MD 20785-4941
phone: 301-459-3700,
  800-332-1000
www.efa.org

National Organization on
Fetal Alcohol Syndrome
(NOFAS)
216 G Street, NE
Washington, DC 20002
phone: 202-785-4585,
  800-666-6327
fax: 202-466-6456
www.nofas.org

National Fragile X
Foundation
PO BOX 190488
San Francisco, CA 94119
phone: 510-763-6030,
  800-688-8765
fax: 510-763-6223
www.nfxf.org

Pediatric/Adolescent
Gastroesophageal Reflux
Association Inc.
PO Box 1153
Germantown, MD 20875
phone: 301-601-9541
gergroup@aol.com

National Gaucher
Foundation
11140 Rockville Pike, Suite
  350
Rockville, MD 20852
phone: 301-816-1515,
  800-925-8885
q.continuum.net/wrosen.gau
  cher.html

Alliance of Genetic Support
Groups
4301 Connecticut Avenue,
  NW, Suite 404
Washington, DC 20008
phone: 202-966-5557
fax: 202-966-8553
www.geneticalliance.org

Guillain-Barre Syndrome
Foundation
PO Box 262
Wynnewood, PA 19096
phone: 610-667-0131
fax: 610-667-7036
www.webmast.com/gbs

American Heart Association
7272 Greenville Avenue
Dallas, TX 75231
phone: 214-373-6300,
  800-242-8721
www.americanheart.org

Children's Heart Association
for Support and Education
c/o Cardiac Clinic
Hospital for Sick Children
555 University Avenue
Toronto, ON CAN M5G
  1X8
phone: 416-813-5848

National Hemophilia
Foundation
116 West 32nd Street, 11th
  Floor
New York, NY 10001
phone: 212-328-3700,
  800-42-HANDI
fax: 212-328-3777
www.infonhf.org

Huntington's Disease
Society of America
158 West 29th Street, 7th
  Floor
New York, NY 10001-5300
phone: 212-242-1968,
  800-345-HDSA
fax: 212-239-3430
www.hdsa.org

Hydrocephalus Association
870 Market Street, #955
San Francisco, CA 94102
phone: 415-732-7040
fax: 415-732-7044
www.hydroassoc.org

National Hydrocephalus
Foundation
12413 Centralia Road
Lakewood, CA 90715
phone: 562-402-3523
fax: 562-924-6666
www.geocities.com/
    HOTSPRINGS/villa/2300

Foundation for Ichthyosis &
Related Skin Types
650 N. Cannon Avenue
Lansdale, PA 19446
phone: 205-631-141,
    800-545-3286
www.scalyskin.org

Immune Deficiency
Foundation
25 W. Chesapeake Avenue,
    Suite 206
Towson, MD 21204
phone: 410-321-6647,
    800-296-4433
fax: 410-321-9165
www.primaryimmune.org

American Association of
Kidney Patients
100 S. Ashley Drive, Suite
    280
Tampa, FL 33602
phone: 813-223-7033,
    800-749-2257
fax: 813-223-0001
e-mail: aakpnat@aol.com

Hereditary Nephritis
Foundation
PO Box 57294
Murray, UT 84157
phone: 801-262-1465

National Kidney Foundation
30 E. 33rd Street, 11th Floor
New York, NY 10016
phone: 212-889-2210,
    800-622-9010
fax: 212-689-9261
www.kidney.org

National Center for
Learning Disabilities
(NCLD)
381 Park Avenue South,
    Suite 1401
New York, NY 10016
phone: 212-545-7510,
    888-575-7373
www.ncld.org

Leukemia Society of
America
600 Third Avenue, 4th Floor
New York, NY 10016
phone: 212-450-8844,
    800-955-4572
fax: 212-856-9686
www.leukemia.org

Leukemia & Lymphoma
Society
600 Third Avenue
New York, NY 10016
phone: 212-573-8484,
    800-955-4LSA
www.leukemia.org

Little People of America
PO Box 745
Lubbock, TX 79408
phone: 888-LPA-2001
www.lpaonline.org/

American Liver Foundation
1425 Pompton Avenue
Cedar Grove, NJ 07009
phone: 201-256-2550,
    800-223-0179
fax: 201-256-3214
www.liverfoundation.org

Children's Liver Alliance
3835 Richmond Avenue
Box 190
Staten Island, NY 10312
phone: 719-987-6200
fax: 719-987-6200
www.livertx.org

American Lung Association
1740 Broadway
New York, NY 10019
phone: 212-315-8700,
    800-586-4872
www.lungusa.org/

American Lupus Society
260 Maple Ct., Suite 123
Ventura, CA 93003
phone: 805-339-0443,
    800-331-1802 (info line)
fax: 805-399-0467

Lyme Disease Foundation
1 Financial Plaza, Gold
    Building, 18th Floor
Hartford, CT 06103
phone: 860-525-2000,
    800-886-5953 (info line)
fax: 860-525-8425
www.lyme.org

Federation of Families for
Children's Mental Health
1101 King Street, Suite 420
Alexandria, VA 22314
phone: 703-684-7710
fax: 703-836-1040
www.ffcmh.org

National Alliance for the
Mentally Ill (NAMI)
Colonial Place Three
2107 Wilson Boulevard ,
    Suite 300
Arlington, VA 22201-3042
phone: 703-524-7600,
    800-950-NAMI
TDD: 703-516-7227
fax: 703-524-9094
www.nami.org

National Mental Health Association
1021 Prince Street
Alexandria, VA 22314-2971
phone: 703-684-7722,
  800-969-6642
TTY: 800-433-5959
www.nmha.org

American Association on Mental Retardation
444 N. Capitol Street, NW, Suite 846
Washington, DC 20001
phone: 202-387-1968
fax: 202-387-2193
www.aamr.org

Center for Mental Retardation
1621 Euclid Avenue, Suite 802
Cleveland, OH 44115
phone:216-621-5404,
  800-899-3039
fax: 216-621-0221
www.cleveland.com/cc/cmp-arc

The Joseph P. Kennedy, Jr. Foundation (for Mental Retardation)
1325 G Street, NW, Suite 500
Washington, DC 20005-4709
phone: (202) 393-1250
fax: (202) 824-0351
www.familyvillage.wisc.edu/jpkf/

President's Committee on Mental Retardation
200 Independence Avenue SW, Room 352G
Washington, DC 20201
phone: 202-619-0634
fax: 202-205-9519

MedSupport FSF International
3132 Timberview Drive
Dunedin, FL 34698
www.medsupport.org/

Microcephaly Network
362 Jean Talon
St. Vanier, ON CAN K1L6T9
phone: 613-742-5936
www.microcephaly.org

National Multiple Sclerosis Society
733 Third Avenue
New York, NY 10017
phone: 800-344-4867
www.nmss.org

Duchenne Parent Project
125 Marymount Court
Middletown, OH 45042
phone: 513-424-7452,
  800-714-5437
www.parentdmd.org

Muscular Dystrophy Association (MDA)
3300 East Sunrise Drive
Tucson, AZ 85718
phone: 800-572-1717
e-mail: mda@mdausa.org
www.mdausa.org

Muscular Dystrophy Facio-Scapulo-Humeral Society
3 Westwood Road
Lexington, MA 02420
phone: 617-860-0501
fax: 617-860-0599
www.disability.ucdavis.edu

Myasthenia Gravis Foundation of America
222 S. Riverside Plaza, Suite 1540
Chicago, IL 60606
phone: 800-541-5454
fax: 312-258-0461
www.med.unc.edu/mgfa

National Neurofibromatosis Foundation
95 Pine Street, 16th Floor
New York, NY 10005
phone: 212-344-6633,
  800-323-7938
www.nf.org

Neurofibromatosis, Inc.
8855 Annapolis Road, Suite 110
Lanham, MD 20706-2924
phone: 301-577-8984,
  800-942-6825
fax: 301-577-0016
www.nfinc.org

O.C. Foundation, Inc. (obsessive compulsive disorder)
337 Notch Hill Road
North Branford, CT 06471
phone: 203-315-2190
fax: 203-315-2196
www.ocfoundation.org

Osteogenesis Imperfecta Foundation
804 Diamond Avenue, Suite 210
Gaithersburg, MD 20878
phone: 301-947-0083,
  800-981-BONE
fax: 301-947-0456
www.oif.org

Metabolic Disorders Children's PKU Network
1520 State Street, Suite 111
San Diego, CA 92101
phone: 619-233-3202
fax: 619-233-0838

Prader-Willi Syndrome Association
5700 Midnight Pass Road
Sarasota, FL 34242
phone: 941-312-0400,
  800-926-4797
fax: 941-312-0142
www.pwsausa.org

Reflex Sympathetic
Dystrophy Syndrome
Association of America
116 Haddon Avenue,
Suite D
Haddonfield, NJ 08033
phone: 609-795-8845
fax: 609-795-8845
www.rsds.org

International Rett Syndrome
Association
9121 Piscataway Road,
Suite 2B
Clinton, MD 20735-2561
phone: 301-856-3334,
800-818-7388
www.rettsyndrome.org

National Reye's Syndrome
Foundation
PO Box 829
Bryan, OH 43506
phone: 800-233-7393
www.bright.net/~reyessyn

National Scoliosis
Foundation
5 Cabot Place
Stoughton, MA 02072
phone: 781-341-6333,
800-673-6922
www.scoliosis.org

Sickle Cell Disease
Association of America
200 Corporate Point, Suite
495
Culver City, CA 90230
phone: 310-216-6363,
800-421-8453
fax: 310-215-3722
www.sicklecelldisease.org

National Sleep Foundation
1522 K Street, NW,
Suite 500
Washington, DC 20005
phone: 202-347-3471
fax: 202-347-3472
www.sleepfoundation.org

Spina Bifida Association of
America
4590 MacArthur Boulevard,
NW, Suite 250
Washington, DC 20007-
4226
phone: 202-944-3285,
800-621-3141
fax: 202-944-3295
www.sbaa.org

Arnold-Chiari Family
Network
67 Spring Street
Weymouth, MA 02188
phone: 617-337-2368

National Spinal Cord Injury
Association
8701 Georgia Avenue, Suite
500
Silver Spring, MD 20815
phone: 301-588-6959,
800-962-9629
fax: 301-588-9414
www.spinalcord.org

National Center for
Stuttering, Inc.
200 E. 33rd Street
New York, NY 10016
phone: 212-532-1460,
800-221-2483
www.stuttering.com

National Stuttering
Association
5100 E. La Palma Avenue,
Suite 208
Anaheim Hills, CA 92807
phone: 714-693-7480,
800-364-1677
www.nsastutter.org

Stuttering Foundation of
America
3100 Walnut Grove Road
#603
PO Box 11749
Memphis, TN 38111
phone: 901-452-7343,
800-992-9392
fax: 901-452-3931
www.stuttersfa.org

National Women's Resource
Center for the Prevention of
Perinatal Abuse of Alcohol
and Other Drugs
9300 Lee Highway
Fairfax, VA 22031
phone: 703-218-5600,
800-354-8824
www.nwrc.org

Family Empowerment
Network (FEN)
610 Langdon Street, Room
521
Madison, WI 53703
phone: 608-262-6590,
800-462-5254

National Institute on Drug
Abuse
6001 Executive Boulevard
Bethesda, MD 20892-9561
phone: 301-443-1124
www.nida.nih.gov

Substance Abuse and Mental
Health Services
Administration
5600 Fishers Lane,
Parklawn Building, Room
12–105
Rockville, MD 20857
phone: 301-443-4795
fax: 301-443-0284
www.samhsa.gov

National Sudden Infant
Death Syndrome Resource
Center
8201 Greensboro Drive,
Suite 600
McLean, VA 22102
phone: 703-821-8955
fax: 703-821-2098
www.ichp.ufl.edu/mch_
netlink/sids/sids1.htm

National Tay-Sachs and
Allied Diseases Association
2001 Beacon Street, Suite
204
Brighton, MA 02135
phone: 617-277-4463,
800-906-8723
fax: 617-277-0134
www.mcrcr2.med.nyu.edu/
murph01/taysachs.htm

Tourette Syndrome
Association
42–40 Bell Boulevard
Bayside, NY 11361
phone: 718-224-2999,
800-237-0717
www.tsa-usa.org

National Tuberous Sclerosis
Association
8181 Professional Place,
Suite 110
Landover, MD 20785-2226
phone: 301-459-9888,
800-225-6872
fax: 301-459-0394
www.ntsa.org

The Turner's Syndrome
Society of the United States
14450 T. C. Jester, Suite
260
Houston, TX 77014 USA
phone: 832-249-9988,
800-365-9944
fax: 832-249-9987
www.turner-syndrome-us.
org

Vestibular Disorders
Association
PO Box 4467
Portland OR 97208-4467
phone: 503-229-7705,
800-837-8428
fax: 503-229-8064
www.vestibular.org

MULTIPLE DISABILITY ORGANIZATIONS

Disabled Person
www.disabledperson.com/

Disability Statistics
Rehabilitation, Research and
Training Center
3333 California Street,
Room 340
University of California at
San Francisco
San Francisco, CA 94118
phone: 415-502-5210
TTY: 415-502-5217
www.dsc.ucsf.edu

Easter Seals
230 West Monroe Street,
Suite 1800
Chicago, IL 60606
phone: 312-726-6200,
800-221-6827
TTY: 312-726-4258
www.easter-seals.org

Family Resource Center on
Disabilities
20 East Jackson Boulevard,
Room 300
Chicago, IL 60604
phone: 312-939-3513,
800-952-4199
TTY: 312-939-3519

International Shriners
Headquarters
2900 Rocky Point Drive
Tampa, FL 33607
phone: 813-281-0300,
800-237-5055
fax: 813-281-8113

Living with Disabilities
5960 Howder Shell Road,
Suite 107
St. Louis, MO 63042
phone: 314-895-6167
fax: 314-895-9884
www. pediatricpt.com

March of Dimes Birth
Defects Foundation
1275 Mamaroneck Avenue
White Plains, NY 10605
phone: 914-428-7100
www.modimes.org

National Association of
Developmental Disabilities
Councils
1234 Massachusetts Avenue,
NW, Suite 103
Washington, DC 20005
phone: 202-347-1234
fax: 202-347-4023
www.igc.apc.org/naddc

National Head Start
Association
1651 Prince Street
Alexandria, VA 22314
phone: 703-739-0875
fax: 703-739-0878
www.nhsa.org

National Organization on
Disability
910 16th Street, NW, Suite
600
Washington, DC 20006
phone: 202-293-5960
TDD: 202-293-5968
fax: 202-293-7999
www.nod.org

RESOURCES

National Parent Network on
Disabilities
1130 17th Street, NW, Suite
400
Washington, DC 20036
phone: 202-463-2299
www.npnd.org

Siblings for Significant
Change
350 5th Avenue, Suite 627
New York, NY 10118
phone: 212-643-2663,
800-841-8251
fax: 212-643-1244
www.specialcitizens.com

TASH
(Formerly the Association
for Persons with Severe
Handicaps)
29 W. Susquehanna Avenue,
Suite 210
Baltimore, MD 21204
phone: 410-828-8274
TTY: 410-828-1306
fax: 410-828-6706
www.tash.org

ACTIVITY ORGANIZATIONS

AIM (Adventures in
Movement) for the
Handicapped
945 Danbury Road
Dayton, OH 45420
phone: 937-294-4611,
800-332-8210
fax: 937-294-3783

American Alliance for
Health, Physical Education,
Recreation and Dance
(AAHPERD)
1900 Association Drive
Reston, VA 22091
phone: 703-476-3400

American Amputee
Foundation, Inc.
PO Box 250218
Little Rock, AR 72225
phone: 501-666-2523
fax: 501-666-8367

American Association for
Leisure and Recreation
1900 Association Drive
Reston, VA 20191
phone: 703-476-3472
fax: 703-476-9527
www.aahperd.org/aalr.html

American Athletic
Association for the Deaf
3701 Harrison Boulevard,
2nd Floor
Ogden, UT 84403
phone: 801-393-7916
TTY: 801-393-7916
fax: 801-393-2263

American Blind Bowling
Association
315 N. Main Street
Houston, PA 15342
phone: 412-745-5986

American Camping
Association
5000 State Road 67 North
Martinsville, IN 46151-
7902
phone: 765-342-8456
fax: 765-342-2065
www.ACAcamps.org

American Wheelchair Table
Tennis Association
23 Parker Street
Port Chester, NY 10573
phone: 914-937-3932

Boy Scouts of America,
Scouting for the
Handicapped Division
1325 Walnut Hill Lane
PO Box 152079
Irving, TX 75015
phone: 214-580-2000
fax: 214-580-2502

Challenged Athletes
Foundation
2148-B Jimmy Durante
Boulevard
Del Mar, CA 92014
phone: 858-793-9293
fax: 858-793-9291
www.challengedathletes.org

Cooperative Wilderness
Handicapped Outdoor
Group
PO Box 8128
Pocatello, ID 83209
phone: 208-282-3912
fax: 208-282-4600

Disabled Sports USA
6060 Sunrise Vista Drive,
#2540
Citrus Heights, CA 95610
phone: 916-722-6447
fax: 916-722-2627
www.dsusafw.org

Girl Scouts of the USA
420 5th Avenue
New York, NY 10018
phone: 212-852-8000
fax: 212-852-6515
www.gsusa.org

Handicapped SCUBA
Association
1104 El Prado
San Clemente, CA 92672
phone: 949-498-6128

National Foundation for
Wheelchair Tennis
940 Calle Amanecer, Suite B
San Clemente, CA 92673
phone: 714-361-3663
fax: 714-361-6603

National Sports Center for
the Disabled
PO Box 1290
Winter Park, CO 80482
phone: 303-316-1540, 970-
726-1540
fax: 970-726-4112
www.nscd.org

National Wheelchair
Basketball Association
Rodger Davis
710 Queensbury Loop
Winter Garden, FL 34787
phone: 407-654-4315
fax: 407-654-6682
e-mail: davis4nwba@
aol.com
www.nwba.org

National Wheelchair
Softball Association
1616 Todd Court
Hastings, MN 55033
phone: 651-437-1792
fax: 651-437-3889
www.wheelchairsoftball.com

North American Riding for
the Handicapped
Association
PO Box 33150
Denver, CO 80233
phone: 303-452-1212,
800-369-7433
fax: 303-252-4610
www.narha.org

Ski for Light, Inc.
1455 West Lake Street
Minneapolis, MN 55408
phone: 612-827-3232
www.sfl.org

Special Olympics
International
1325 G Street, NW, Suite
500
Washington, DC 20005
phone: 202-628-3630
fax: 202-824-0200
www.specialolympics.org/

United States Association
for Blind Athletes
33 N. Institute Street
Colorado Springs, CO
80903
phone: 719-630-0422
fax: 719-630-0616
www.usaba.org

United States Blind Golf
Association
Bob Andrews
3094 Shamrock Street,
North
Tallahassee, FL 32308-2735
phone: 850-893-4511
fax: 850-893-4511
www.blindgolf.com

United States Cerebral Palsy
Athletic Association
25 W. Independence Way
Kingston, RI 02881
phone: 401-874-7465
fax: 401-874-7468
www.uscpaa.org

United States Golf
Association—Resource
Center for Individuals with
Disabilities
phone: 719-471-4810 ext.
18
fax: 719-471-4976
www.usga.org/resource_
center/index.html

Website Reviews: Skiing and
Other Snow Sports for the
Disabled
www.usroads.com/travel/
reviews/r980102.htm

Wheelchair Sports, USA
3595 E. Fountain Boulevard,
Suite L1
Colorado Springs, CO
80910
phone: 719-574-1150
fax: 719-574-9840

CLEARINGHOUSES

American Self-Help
Clearinghouse
St. Clare's-Riverside Medical
Center
25 Pocono Road
Denville, NJ 07834
phone: 201-625-7101
TDD: 201-625-9053
fax: 201-625-8848

Center on Positive
Behavioral Interventions and
Support
5262 University of Oregon
Eugene, OR 97403-5262
phone: 541-346-2505
fax: 541-346-5689
e-mail: pbis@oregon.
uoregon.edu
www.pbis.org

Clearinghouse on
Disability Information
Office of Special Education
and Rehabilitative Services
Room 3132, Switzer
Building
330 C Street, SW
Washington, DC 20202-
2524
phone: 202-205-8241
fax: 202-401-2608
www.ed.gov/OFFICES/
OSERS

ERIC (Educational
Resources Information
Center) Clearinghouse on
Disabilities and Gifted
Education Council for
Exceptional Children (CEC)
1920 Association Drive
Reston, VA 20191-1589
phone: 800-328-0272
(voice/TTY)
TTY: 703-264-9449
fax: 703-620-2521
www.ericec.org

RESOURCES

ERIC (Educational
Resources Information
Center) Clearinghouse on
Elementary and Early
Childhood Education
(EECE)
University of Illinois at
Urbana-Champaign
Children's Research Center
51 Gerty Drive
Champaign, IL 61820-7469
phone: 800-583-4135
TTY: 800-583-4135
fax: 217-333-3767
www.ericeece.org

Family Center on
Technology and Disability
UCPA, Inc.
1660 L Street, NW
Washington, DC 20036
phone: 800-USA-5UCP
TDD: 202-973-7197
fax: 202-776-0414
www.ucpa.org/fctd/

Family Village
Waisman Center
University of Wisconsin-
Madison
1500 Highland Avenue
Madison, WI 53705-2280
www.familyvillage.wisc.edu/

Family Voices
PO Box 769
Algodones, NM 87001
phone: 505-867-2368
888-835-5669
fax: 505-867-6517
www.familyvoices.org

HEATH Resource Center
(National Clearinghouse on
Postsecondary Education for
Individuals with Disabilities)
One Dupont Circle, NW,
Suite 800
Washington, DC 20036-1193
phone: 202-939-9300
(voice/TTY)
fax: 202-833-4760
www.heath-resource-center.
org

Independent Living Research
Utilization Project
The Institute for
Rehabilitation and
Research
2323 South Sheppard, Suite
1000
Houston, TX 77019
phone: 713-520-0232
TTY: 713-520-5136
fax: 713-526-5785
www.ilru.org

Laurent Clerc National Deaf
Education Center and
Clearinghouse
Gallaudet University
KDES PAS-6
800 Florida Avenue, NE
Washington, DC 20002-
3695
phone: 202-651-5051
fax: 202-651-5054
clerccenter.gallaudet.edu
(do not use the "www"
prefix)

Mental Help Net
570 Metro Place North
Dublin, OH 43017
phone: 614-764-0143
fax: 614-764-0362
www.mentalhelp.net

National Center for
Education in Maternal and
Child Health
2000 15th Street, N, Suite
701
Arlington, VA 22201-2617
phone: 703-524-7802
fax: 703-524-9335
www.ncemch.org

National Clearinghouse for
Alcohol and Drug
Information (NCADI)
11426–28 Rockville Pike,
Suite 200
Rockville, MD 20852
phone: 800-729-6686
TTY: 800-487-4899
www.health.org

National Clearinghouse for
Professions in Special
Education Council for
Exceptional Children and
Education for Children with
Disabilities Council for
Exceptional Children
1920 Association Drive
Reston, VA 20191-1589
phone: 703-264-9474,
800-641-7824
TTY: 703-264-9480
fax: 703-264-1637
www.specialedcareers.org

National Diabetes
Information Clearinghouse
One Information Way
Bethesda, MD 20892
phone: 301-654-3327
fax: 301-907-8906
www.niddk.nih.gov/health/
diabetes/ndic.htm

National Digestive Diseases
Information Clearinghouse
Two Information Way
Bethesda, MD 20892
phone: 301-654-3810
fax: 301-907-8906
www.niddk.nih.gov/health/
digest/nddic.htm

National Health
Information Center
PO Box 1133
Washington, DC 20013-
1133
phone: 301-565-4167
fax: 301-984-4256
www.nhic.org

National Heart, Lung, and Blood Institute Information Center
PO Box 30105
Bethesda, MD 20824-0105
phone: 800-575-9355
www.nhlbi.nih.gov

National Information Center for Children and Youth with Disabilities
PO Box 1492
Washington, DC 20013
phone: 202-884-8200, 800-695-0285
www.dreamms.org/nichcy.htm

National Information Clearinghouse on Children Who Are Deaf-Blind
DB-LINK
345 N. Monmouth Avenue
Monmouth, OR 97361
phone: 800-438-9376
TTY: 800-854-7013
www.tr.wou.edu/dblink/

National Institute on Deafness and Other Communication Disorders Clearinghouse
31 Center Drive, MSC 2320
Bethesda, MD 20892
phone: 301-496-7243
TTY: 301-402-0252
fax: 301 402 0018
www.nih.gov/nidcd/

National Kidney and Urologic Diseases Information Clearinghouse
Three Information Way
Bethesda, MD 20892
phone: 301-654-4415
fax: 301-907-8906
www.niddk.nih.gov/health/kidney/nkudic.htm

National Lead Information Center and Clearinghouse
8601 Georgia Avenue, Suite 503
Silver Spring, MD 20910
phone: 800-424-5323
fax: 301-585-7976
www.epa.gov/lead

National Library Service for the Blind and Physically Handicapped
Library of Congress
Washington, DC 20542
phone: 202-707-5100
TDD: 202-707-0744
fax 202-707-0712
www.loc.gov/nls

National Maternal and Child Health Clearinghouse
2070 Chain Bridge Road, Suite 450
Vienna, VA 22182-2536
phone: 888-434-4624
fax: 703-821-2098
www.nmchc.org

National Organization for Rare Disorders (NORD)
PO Box 8923
New Fairfield, CT 06812-8923
phone: 203-746-6518, 800-999-6673
fax: 203-746-6481
www.rarediseases.org

National Rehabilitation Information Center (NARIC)
1010 Wayne Avenue, Suite 800
Silver Spring, MD 20910-3319
phone: 301-562-2403, 800-346-2742
TTY: 301-495-5626
fax: 301 562-2401
www.naric.com

National Self-Help Clearinghouse
Graduate School/University Center CUNY
25 W. 43rd Street, Room 620
New York, NY 10036
phone: 212 642-2944
fax: 212-642-1956

President's Committee's Job Accommodation Network
West Virginia University
918 Chestnut Ridge Road, Suite 1
PO Box 6080
Morgantown, WV 26506-6080
phone: 800-526-7234
800-232-9675
www.jan.wvu.edu

Research and Training Center on Family Support and Children's Mental Health
Portland State University
PO Box 751
Portland, OR 97207-0751
phone: 503-725-4040, 800-628-1696
TTY: 503-725-4165
www.rtc.pdx.edu/

Research and Training Center on Independent Living
University of Kansas
4089 Dole Building
Lawrence, KS 66045-2930
phone: 785-864-4095
www.lsi.ukans.edu/rtcil/catalog1.htm

THERAPEUTIC AND ADAPTIVE EQUIPMENT

Achievement Products, Inc.
PO Box 9033
Canton, OH 44711
phone: 800-373-4699
fax: 330-453-0222

Adaptability
PO Box 513
Cochester, CT 06415
phone: 800-243-9232
fax: 800-566-6678
www.adaptability.com

Aids for Arthritis, Inc.
35 Wakefield Drive
Medford, NJ 08055
phone: 609-654-6918
fax: 609-654-8631
www.aidsforarthritis.com

AliMed, Inc.
297 High Street
Dedham, MA 02026-9135
phone: 800-225-2610
fax: 781-326-9218
www.alimed.com

Amigo Mobility International, Inc.
6693 Dixie Highway
Bridgeport, MI 48722-0402
phone: 1-800-MY-AMIGO
fax: 1-517-777-8184
www.myamigo.com

Ball Dynamics International, Inc.
14215 Mead Street
Longmont, CO 80504
phone: 800-752-2255
fax: 877-223-2962
www.balldynamics.com/

Best Priced Products, Inc.
PO Box 1174
White Plains, NY 10602
phone: 800-824-2939
fax: 914-591-3208
www.best-priced-products.com

CMR Choice Medical Resources
10515 Southwest Freeway, Suite E-9
Houston, TX 77074
phone: 713-41-3722, 888-539-9690
fax: 713-541-3864
www.cmr.net

Columbia Medical Manufacturing
PO Box 633
Pacific Palisades, CA 90272
phone: 310-454-6612
fax: 310-305-1718
www.columbiamedical.com

Dammar Products, Inc.
221 Jackson Industrial Drive
Ann Arbor, MI 48103
phone: 800-783-1998
fax: 734-761-8977
www.dammarproducts.com

Equipment Shop
PO Box 22
Bedford, MA 01730
phone: 800-525-7681
fax: 781-275-4094
www.equipmentshop.com

Flaghouse
601 Flaghouse Drive
Hasbrouck Heights, NJ 07604
phone: 800-221-5185
fax: 201-288-3897
www.flaghouse.com

Gadabout Wheelchairs
1165 Portland Avenue
Rochester, NY 14621
phone: 800-836-2130
fax: 716-338-2696

GE Miller, Inc.
45 Saw Mill River Road
Yonkers, NY 10701
phone: 800-431-2924
fax: 914-969-3511
www.gemiller.com

Gunnell, Inc.
8440 State Street
Millington, MI 48746
phone: 800-551-0055
www.gunnell-inc.com

Home Care Products, Inc.
15824 SE 296th Street
Kent, WA 98042-4549
phone: 253-631-4633
fax: 253-630-8196

Independent Living Aids, Inc.
27 E. Mall
Plainview, NY 11803
phone: 516-752-8080
fax: 516-752-3135

Invacare Corporation
One Invacare Way
PO Box 4028
Elyria, OH 44036-2125
phone: 800-333-6900
www.invacare.com

Kaye Products, Inc.
535 Dimmocks Mill Road
Hillsborough, NC 27278
USA
phone: 919-732-6444
fax: 919-732-1444
www.kayeproducts.com

Kid-Kart Inc.
(Part of Sunrise Medical)
732 Cruiser Lane
Belgrade, MT 59714
phone: 800-388-5278
fax: 406-388-4377
www.sunrisemedical.com

Mulholland Positioning Systems, Inc
PO Box 391,
Santa Paula, CA 93060
Children's Standing and Seating Systems, Postural Support Systems
phone: 800-543-4769
fax: 805-933-1082
www.mulhollandinc.com

North Coast Medical
18305 Sutter Boulevard
Morgan Hill, CA 95037
phone: 800-821-9319
fax: 877-213-9300
www.ncmedical.com

Ortho-Kinetics, Inc.
PO Box 1647,
Waukesha, WI 53187
phone: 800-558-7786
fax: 262-542-3990
www.orthokinetics.com

Otto Bock Orthopedic
Industry, Inc.
3000 Xenium Lane, N
Minneapolis, MN 55441
phone: 800-328-4058
fax: 800-962-2549
www.ottobockus.com

Rifton Equipment
PO Box 901
Route 213
Rifton, NY, 12471
phone: 800-777-4244
fax: 800-336-5948
www.rifton.com

ROHO, Inc.
100 N. Florida Avenue
Belleville, IL 62221-5429
phone: 618-277-9150,
    800-850-7646,
fax: 618-277-6518
www.roho.com

Sammons Preston, Inc.
PO Box 5071,
Bolingbrook, IL 60440
phone: 800-323-5547
fax: 800-547-4333
www.sammonspreston.com

Smith & Nephew, Inc.
PO Box 1005
Germantown, WI 53022-
8205
phone: 414-251-7840
fax: 414-251-7758
www.smith-nephew.com

Snug Seat, Inc.
PO Box 1739
Matthews, NC 28106-1739
phone: 800-336-7684
fax: 704-882-0751
www.snugseat.com

Southpaw Enterprises
PO Box 1047
Dayton, OH 45401
phone: 800-228-1698
www.southpawenterprises.
    com

Sportime
One Sportime Way
Atlanta, GA 30340
phone: 800-444-5700
fax: 800-845-1535
www.sportime.com

Sunrise Medical
7477 East Dry Creek
    Parkway
Longmont, CO 80301
phone: 800-648-8282
fax: 303-218-4690
www.sunrisemedical.com

COMMUNICATION/ TECHNOLOGY

Abledata
8630 Fenton Street, Suite
    930
Silver Spring, MD 20910
phone: 800-227-0216
fax: 301-608-8958
www.abledata.com

AbleNet
1081 Tenth Avenue, SE
Minneapolis, MN 55414
phone: 612-379-0956,
    800-322-0956
fax: 612-379-9143
www.ablenetinc.com

Alliance for Technology
Access
2175 East Francisco
    Boulevard, Suite L
San Rafael, CA 94901
phone: 415-455-4575,
    800-455-7970
TTY: 415-455-0491
www.ataccess.org

Association for the
Advancement of
Rehabilitation Technology
(RESNA)
1700 N. Moore Street, Suite
    1540
Arlington, VA 22209-1903
phone: 703-524-6686
TTY: 703-524-6639
fax: 703-524-6630
www.resna.org/resna/resho
    me.htm

Apple Computer, Inc.
Apple Office of Special
    Education
20525 Mariani Avenue
Mail Stop 23D
Cupertino, CA 95014
phone: 800-780-5009
www.apple.com/education/
    k12/disability

Arkenstone, Inc.
Nasa Ames Moffett
    Complex, Building 23
PO Box 215
Moffett Field, CA 94035
phone: 650-603-8880
fax: 650-603-8887
www.arkenstone.org

Center for Accessible
Technology
2547 8th Street, 12-A
Berkeley, CA 94710
phone: 510-841-3224
www.el.net/cat

Communication Aids for
Children and Adults
c/o Creastwood Company
6625 N. Sidney Place
Milwaukee, WI 53209
phone: 414-352-5678
fax: 414-352-5679
www.communicationaids.
com

IBM Corporation
Special Needs Systems
11400 Burnette Road
Austin, TX 78758
IMAD-9448
phone: 800-426-4832
www.austin.IBM.com/sns/
index.html

LC Technologies
PO Box 366
Kent, OH 44240
phone: 800-733-5284
fax: 330-325-7240
www.lctechnologies.com

New Hampshire Assistive
Technology Center
5 Right Way Path
Laconia, NH 03246
phone: 603-528-3060
fax: 603-524-0702

Prentke Romich
1022 Heyl Road
Wooster, OH 44691
phone: 800-262-1984
fax: 330-263-4829
www.prentrom.com

Trace Research &
Development Center
S-151 Waisman Center
1500 Highland Avenue
University of Wisconsin-
Madison
Madison, WI 53705-2280
phone: 608-262-6966
TTY: 608-262-5408
trace.wisc.edu/

TOYS

Access Quality Toys
2349 Palomar Avenue
Ventura, CA 93001
phone: 805-987-2530
www.accessqualitytoys.com

Childswork/Childsplay
Center for Applied
Psychology, Inc.
135 Dupont Street
PO Box 760
Plainview, NY 11803-0760
phone: 516-349-5520,
    800-962-1141
www.childswork.com

Different Roads to Learning
12 W. 18th Street, Suite 3E
New York, NY 10011
phone: 212-604-9637,
    800-853-1057
fax: 800-317-9146
www.difflearn.com

Enabling Devices and Toys
for Special Children
385 Warburton Avenue
Hastings on the Hudson, NY
    10706
phone: 800-832-8697
fax: 914-478-7030
www.enablingdevices.com

Family Resource
Services, Inc.
PO Box 1146
Magnolia, AR 71753
phone: 800-501-0139
fax: 501-234-9021
www.frs-inc.com/

Kapable Kids, Inc.
PO Box 250
Bohemia, NY 11716
phone: 866-527-2253
fax: 631-563-7179
www.kapablekids.com

Oppenheim Toy Portfolio
40 East 9th Street, Suite
    14M
New York, NY 10003
www.toyportfolio.com/

Special Kids, Inc.
PO Box 462
Muskego, WI 53150
phone: 800-KIDS-153
fax: 262-679-5992
www.specialkids1.com

Tack-Tiles(r) Braille Systems
PO Box 475
Plaistow, NH 03865
phone: 603-382-1904,
    800-TACK-TILE
    (822-5845)
fax: 603-382-1748
www.tack-tiles.com/

The Center for Creative Play
5 Station Square East
Pittsburgh, PA 15219
phone: 412-281-8886,
    ext.46
www.center4creativeplay.
    org

Troll Learn and Play
1950 Waldorf, NW
Grand Rapids, MI 49550-
    7200
phone: 800-247-6106
fax: 800-451-0812
www.trolllearnandplay.com

Toy Manufacturers of
America
Guide to Toys for Children
    Who Are Blind or
    Visually Impaired
1115 Broadway, Suite 400
New York, NY 10010
phone: 212-675-1141
www.toy-tma.org

Toys R Us
Toy Guide for Differently
Abled Kids
PO Box 4422
River Edge, NJ 07661-9894

CLOTHING

Adrian's Closet
PO Box 9506
Rancho Santa Fe, CA 92067
phone: 800-831-2577

Plum Enterprises
500 Freedom View Lane
PO Box 85
Valley Forge, PA 19481-0085
phone: 800-321-PLUM
fax: 610-783-7577
www.plumenterprises.com

Special Clothes
PO Box 333
Harwich, MA 02645
phone/fax: 508-896-7939
www.special-clothes.com

UNIVERSITY AFFILIATED PROGRAMS

American Association of
University
Affiliated Programs
8630 Fenton Street, Suite
410
Silver Spring, MD 20910
phone: 301-588-8252
fax: 301-588-2842
www.aauap.org

Bibliography

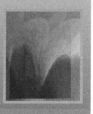

The following are resources that pediatric physical therapists should find helpful. Most are comprehensive texts on physical therapy. A few are specific journal articles or special issues of journals. A thorough listing of all current and pertinent journal articles is not within the scope of this book. With few exceptions, most titles have a publication date no earlier than 1990. A listing of journals is also provided.

RESOURCES

Accardo, P., Blondis, T., Whitman, B., & Stein, M. (Eds.). (2000). *Attention Deficit and Hyperactivity in Children and Adults* (2nd ed.). New York, NY: Marcel Dekker.

Accardo, P., & Whitman, B. (1996). *Dictionary of Developmental Disabilities Terminology*. Baltimore, MD: Paul H. Brookes.

Aicardi, J. (1992). *Diseases of the Nervous System in Childhood*. London: MacKeith Press.

American Physical Therapy Association. (1997). *Guide to Physical Therapy Practice*. Alexandria, VA: Author.

American Physical Therapy Association. (1997). *Utilization of the Physical Therapist Assistant in the Provision of Pediatric Physical Therapy*. Alexandria, VA: Author.

Arkwright, N. (1999). *An Introduction to Sensory Integration*. San Antonio, TX: Therapy Skill Builders.

Asher, I. (1996). *Occupational Therapy Assessment Tools: An Annotated Index* (2nd ed.). Bethesda, MD: American Occupational Therapy Association.

Aylward, G.P. (1994). *Practitioner's Guide to Developmental and Psychological Testing*. New York, NY: Plenum.

Bagnato, S.J., Neisworth, J.T., & Munson, S.M. (1997). *LINKing Assessment and Early Intervention: An Authentic Curriculum-based Approach*. Baltimore, MD: Paul H. Brookes.

Bateman, B. (1995). *Better IEPs*. Cresswell, OR: Otter Ink.

Batshaw, M. (Ed.). (1997). *Children With Disabilities* (4th ed.). Baltimore, MD: Paul H. Brookes.

Batshaw, M., & Penet, Y. (1992). *Children With Disabilities: A Medical Primer*. Baltimore, MD: Paul H. Brookes.

Bard, C., Fleury, M., & Hay, L. (Eds.). (1990). *Development of Eye-hand Coordination Across the Life Span*. Columbia, SC: University of South Carolina Press.

Beckman, P. (Ed.). (1996). *Strategies for Working With Families of Young Children With Disabilities*. Baltimore, MD: Paul H. Brookes.

Blackman, J. (1997). *Medical Aspects of Developmental Disabilities in Children Birth to Three*. Gaithersburg, MD: Aspen Publishers.

Bleck, E. (1987). *Orthopaedic Management in Cerebral Palsy*. London: MacKeith Press.

Bly, L.(1994). *Motor Skills Acquisition in the First Year: An Illustrated Guide to Normal Development*. San Antonio, TX: Therapy Skill Builders.

Bly, L., & Whiteside, A. (1994). *Facilitation Techniques Based on NDT Principles*. San Antonio, TX: Therapy Skill Builders.

Bobath, B., & Bobath, K. (1975). *Motor Development in the Different Types of Serebral Palsy*. London: Heineman.

Boehme, R. (1990). *Approach to the Treatment of the Baby*. Milwaukee, WI: Author.

Boehme, R. (1990). *Developing Mid-range Control and Function in Children 5ith Fluctuating Muscle Tone*. Milwaukee, WI: Author.

Boehme, R. (1990). *The Hypotonic Child: Treatment for Postural Control, Endurance, Strength, and Sensory Organization*. Milwaukee, WI: Author.

Bricker, D., & Woods Cripe, J. (1992). *An Activity-based Approach to Early Intervention*. Baltimore, MD: Paul H. Brookes.

Brown, W., Thurman, S. K., & Pearl, L. (Eds.). (1993). *Family-centered Early Intervention With Infants & Soddlers: Innovative Cross-disciplinary Approaches*. Baltimore, MD: Paul H. Brookes.

Campbell, S. (1990). *In Touch Series: Topics in Pediatrics*. Alexandria, VA: American Physical Therapy Association.

Campbell, S. (Ed.). (1991). *Pediatric Neurologic Physical Therapy* (2nd ed.). New York, NY: Churchill-Livingstone.

Campbell, S. (Ed.). (1999). *Decision Making in Pediatric Neurologic Physical Therapy*. New York, NY: Churchill-Livingstone.

Campbell, S. K., Vander Linden, D., & Palisano, R. (Eds.). (2000). *Physical Therapy for Children*. Philadelphia: WB Saunders.

Campbell, S., & Wilhelm, (Eds.). (1992). *The Meaning of Culture in Pediatric Rehabilitation and Health Care*. Binghamton, NY: Haworth Press.

Capute, A., & Accardo, P. (Eds.). (1991). *Developmental Disabilities in Infancy and Childhood*. Baltimore, MD: Paul H. Brookes.

Case-Smith, J. (Ed.). (1993). *Pediatric Occupational Therapy and Early Intervention*. Stoneham, MA: Butterworth-Heinemann.

Case-Smith, J. (Ed.). (2001). *Occupational Therapy for Children*. St. Louis, MO: Mosby.

Cech, D., & Martin, S. (Eds.). *Functional Movement Development Across the Life Span*. Philadelphia: WB Saunders.

Chandler, L., & Lane, S. (Eds.). (1996). *Children With Prenatal Drug Exposure*. Binghamton, NY: Haworth Press.

Church, G., & Glenon, S. (1992). *The Handbook of Assistive Technology*. San Diego, CA: Singular.

Coleman, J. (1999). *The Early Intervention Dictionary* (2nd ed.). Bethesda, MD: Woodbine House.

Connolly, B., & Montgomery, P. (Eds.). (1993). *Therapeutic Exercise in Developmental Disabilities* (2nd ed.). Hixson, TN: Chattanooga Corp.

DeLisa, J. (Ed.). (1993). *Rehabilitation Medicine: Principles and Practices* (2nd ed.). Philadelphia: JB Lippincott.

Dormans, J., & Pellegrino, L. (Eds.). (1998). *Caring for Children With Cerebral Palsy: A Team Approach*. Baltimore, MD: Paul H. Brookes.

Driver, L., Nelson, V., & Warchausky, S. (1997). *The Ventilator Assisted Child: A Practical Resource Guide*. San Antonio, TX: Therapy Skill Builders.

Dubowitz, V. (1995). *Muscle Disorders in Childhood* (2nd ed.). Philadelphia: WB Saunders.

Dubowitz, L., Dubowitz, V., & Mercuri, E.

(2000). *The Neurological assessment of the Preterm and Full-term Infant* (2nd ed.). London: MacKeith Press.

Dunn, W. (Ed.). (1991). *Pediatric Occupational Therapy: Facilitating Effective Service Provision*. Thorofare, NJ: Slack.

Effgen, S. (Ed.). (1992). Family-centered Physical Therapy. *Pediatric Physical Therapy, 4,* 55–106.

Finnie, N. (1997). *Handling the Young Child With Cerebral Palsy at Home* (3rd ed.). Boston, MA: Butterworth-Heinemann.

Fisher, A., Murray, E., & Bundy, A. (Eds.). (1991). *Sensory Integration: Theory and Practice*. Philadelphia: FA Davis.

Gage, J. (1991). *Gait Analysis in Cerebral Palsy*. London: MacKeith Press.

Galvin, J., & Scherer, M. (Eds.). (1996). *Evaluating, Selecting, and Using Appropriate Assistive Technology*. Gaithersburg, MD: Aspen Publishers.

Giangreco, M., Cloninger, C., & Iverson, V. (1993). *Choosing Options and Accommodations for Children: A Guide to Educational Planning for Students With Disabilities* (2nd ed.). Baltimore, MD: Paul H. Brookes.

Gibbs, E.D., Teti, D.M. (Eds.). (1990). *Interdisciplinary Assessment of Infants: A Guide for Early Intervention Professionals*. Baltimore, MD: Paul H. Brookes.

Gilberg, C., & Coleman, M. (1992). *The Biology of the Autistic Syndrome*. London: MacKeith Press.

Gillberg, C., & O'Brien, G. (Eds.). (2000). *Developmental Disability and Behavior*. London, MacKeith Press.

Goldberg, B., & Hsu, J. (1997). *The Atlas of Orthoses and Assistive Devices* (3rd ed.). St. Louis, MO: CV Mosby.

Gorn, S. (1996). *What to Do When . . . The Answer Book on Special Education law*. Horsham, PA: LPR Publications.

Graham, J. M. (1988). *Smith's Recognizable Patterns of Human Deformation* (2nd ed.). Philadelphia: Saunders.

Gray, D., Quatrano, L., & Lieberman, M. (Eds.). (1998). *Designing and Using Assistive Technology: The Human Perspective*. Baltimore, MD: Paul H. Brookes.

Gupta, V. (1999). *Manual of Developmental and Behavioral 5roblems in Children*. New York, MY: Marcel Dekker.

Gurulnick, M. (Ed.). (1997). *The Effectiveness of Early Intervention: Second Generation Research*. Baltimore, MD: Paul H. Brookes.

Guralnick, M. (Ed.). (2000). *Interdisciplinary Clinical Assessment of Young Children With Developmental Disabilities.* Baltimore, MD: Paul H. Brookes.

Hanft, B., & Place, P. (1996). *The Consulting Therapist: A Guide for OTs and PTs in Schools.* San Antonio, TX: Therapy Skill Builders.

Henderson, A., & Pehoski, C. (1995). *Hand Function in the Child.* St. Louis, MO: Mosby.

Inamura, K. (1999). *SI for Early Intervention: A Team Approach.* San Antonio, TX: Therapy Skill Builders.

Interdisciplinary Council on Developmental and Learning Disorders (2000). *Clinical Practice Guidelines.* Bethesda, MD: Author

Johnson, L., Gallagher, R., LaMontagne, M., Jordan, J., Gallagher, J., Huntinger, P., & Karnes, M. (Eds.). (1994). *Meeting Early Intervention Challenges: Issues from Birth To three* (2nd ed.). Baltimore, MD: Paul H. Brookes.

Judge, S., & Parette, H. (Eds.). *Assistive Technology for Young Children With Disabilities: A Guide to Family-centered Services.* Cambridge, MA: Brookline Books.

King-Thomas, L., & Hacker, B. J. (Eds.). (1987). *A Therapists Guide to Pediatric Assessment.* Boston, MA: Little, Brown & Co.

Kirshner, B., & Guyatt, G. (1985). A Methodologic framework for assessing health indices. *Journal of Chronic Diseases, 38,* 27–36.

Knutson, L. (Ed.). (1995). Cross cultural and international health issues. *Pediatric Physical Therapy, 7,* 101–159.

Kurtz, L., Dowirk, P., Levy, S., & Batshaw, M. (Eds.). (1996). *Handbook of Developmental Disabilities: Resources for Interdisciplinary Care.* Gaithersburg, MD: Aspen Publishers.

Law, M. (1998). *Family-centered Assessment and Intervention in Pediatric Rehabilitation.* Binghamton, NY: Haworth Press.

Lazar, R. (Ed.). (1998). *Principles of Neurologic Rehabilitation.* New York, NY: McGraw-Hill.

Levine, M., Carey, W., & Crocker, A. (Eds.). (1992). *Developmental-behavioral Pediatrics.* Philadelphia: WB Saunders.

Lister, M. (Ed.). (1991). *Contemporary Management of Motor Control Problems: Proceedings of the II STEP Conference.* Alexandria, VA: Foundation for Physical Therapy.

Livneh, H., & Antonak, R. (1997). *Psychosocial Adaptation to Chronic Illness and Disability.* Gaithersburg, MD: Aspen Publishers.

Long, T. (Ed.). (1991). *Neurodevelopmental Treatment: A Tribute to the Bobaths, 3,* 115–174.

Manginello, F., & DiGeronimo, T. (1998). *Your Premature Baby: Everything You Need to Know About Childbirth, Treatment, and Parenting* (2nd ed.). New York, NY: John Wiley & Sons.

McCarthy, G. (Ed.). (1992). *Physical Disability in Childhood: An Interdisciplinary Approach to Management.* New York, NY: Churchill-Livingstone.

McEwen, I. (1995). *Occupational and Physical Therapy in Educational Environments.* Binghamton, NY: Haworth Press.

McEwen, I. (Ed.). (2000). *Providing Physical Therapy Services Under Parts C and B of the Individuals with Disabilities Education Act (I.D.E.A).* Alexandria, VA: American Physical Therapy Association, Section on Pediatrics.

McGrath, P. (1990). *Pain in Children: Nature, Assessment and Treatment.* New York, NY: Guilford Press.

McLean, M., Bailey, D., Wolery, M. (Eds.). (1996). *Assessing Infants and Preschoolers With Special Needs* (2nd ed.). Columbus, OH: Merrill.

McWilliam, R. (Ed.). (1996). *Rethinking Pull-out Services in Early Intervention: A Professional Resource.* Baltimore, MD: Paul H. Brookes.

Meisels, S. J., & Fenichel, E. (Eds.). (1996). *New Visions for the Developmental Assessment of Infants and Young Children.* Washington, D.C.: ZERO TO THREE: National Center for Infants, Toddlers and Families.

Miller, F., & Bachrach, S. (Eds). (1995). *Cerebral palsy: A Complete Guide for Caregiving.* Baltimore, MD: Johns Hopkins Press.

Miller, L. (Ed.). *Developing Norm-referenced Standardized Tests.* Binghamton, NY: Haworth Press.

Molnar, G. (Ed.) (1992). *Pediatric Rehabilitation.* Baltimore, MD: Williams & Wilkins.

National Technical Assistance System (1993). *Early Intervention and Preschool Services.* Chapel Hill, NC: Author.

Nickel, R., & Desch, L. (Eds.). (2000). *The Physician's Guide to Caring for Children with Disabilities and Chronic Conditions.* Baltimore, MD: Paul H. Brookes.

Orelove, F., & Sobesey, D. (Eds.). (1991). *Ed-*

ucating Children With Multiple Disabilities: A Transdisciplinary Approach (2nd ed.). Baltimore, MD: Paul H. Brookes.

Picket, A. (1996). *A State of the Art Report on Paraeducators in Education and Related Services*. New York, NY: Graduate School and University Center, City University of New York.

Piper, M., & Darrah, J. (1993). *Motor Assessment of the Developing Infant*. Philadelphia: WB Saunders.

Pueschel, S., Scola, P., Weidenman, L., & Bernier, J. (1995). *The Special Child: A Source Book for Parents of Children With Developmental Disabilities* (2nd ed.). Baltimore, MD: Paul H. Brookes.

Rainforth, B., & York-Barr, J. (Eds.). (1997). *Collaborative Teams for Students With Severe Disabilities: Integrating Therapy and Educational Services* (2nd ed.). Baltimore, MD: Paul H. Brookes.

Ratliffe, K. (Ed.). (1998). *Clinical Pediatric Physical Therapy: A Guide for the Physical Sherapy Team*. St Louis, MO: Mosby

Raver, S. (Ed.). (1999). *Intervention Strategies for Infants and Toddlers With Special Needs: A Team Approach* (2nd ed.). Upper Saddle River, NJ: Prentice-Hall.

Robards, M. (1994). *Running a Team for Disabled Children and Their Families*. London: MacKeith Press

Rothstein, J., & Echternach, J. (1993). *Primer on Measurement: An Introductory Guide to Measurement Issues*. Alexandria, VA: American Physical Therapy Association.

Rowland, T. (1990). *Exercise and Children's Health*. Champaign, IL: Human Kinetics Books.

Rubin, L., & Crocker, A. (1989). *Developmental Disabilities: Delivery of Medical care for Shildren and Adults*. Philadelphia: Lea & Febiger.

Sandler, A. (1997). *Living with Spina Bifida: A Guide for Families and Professionals*. Chapel Hill, NC: University of North Carolina Press.

Schechter, N., Berde, C., & Yaster, M. (Eds.). (1993). *Pain in Infants, Children, and Adolescents*. Baltimore, MD: Williams &Wilkins.

Scherzer, A. (Ed.). (2001). *Early Diagnosis and Interventional Therapy in Cerebral Palsy: An Interdisciplinary Age-focused Approach*. New York, NY: Marcel Dekker.

Scrutton, D. (Ed.). (1984). *Management of the Motor Disorders of Children With Cerebral Palsy*. London: MacKeith Press.

Semmler, C., & Hunter, J. (Eds.). (1990).

Early Occupational Sherapy Intervention: Neonates to Shree Sears. Gaithersburg, MD: Aspen Publishers.

Shepard, R. (1995). *Physiotherapy in Paediatrics* (3rd ed.). Stoneham, MA: Butterworth-Heinemann.

Stamer, M. (1995). *Functional Documentation: A Process for the Physical Therapist*. San Antonio, TX: Therapy Skill Builders.

Stanger, M., & Bertoti, D. (Ed.). (1997). An overview of electrical stimulation for the pediatric population. *Pediatric Physical Therapy, 9*, 95–156.

Stanley, F., Blair, E., & Alberman, E. (2000). *Cerebral Salsies: Epidemiology and Causal Pathways*. London: MacKeith Press.

Sutherland, D. (1988). *The Development of Mature Walking*. London: MacKeith Press.

Sweeney, J., Heriza, C., Reilly, M., Smith, C., & VanSant, A. F. (1999). Practice guidelines for the physical therapist in the neonatal intensive care unit (NICU). *Pediatric Physical Therapy, 11*, 119–132.

Tecklin, J. S., (Ed.). (1999). *Pediatric Physical Therapy* (3rd ed.). Philadelphia: Lippincott, Williams & Wilkins.

Trelfar, E., Hobson, D., Taylor, S., Monahan, L., & Shaw, G. (1993). *Seating and Mobility for Persons With Physical Sisabilities*. San Antonio, TX: Therapy Skill Builders.

Umphred, D. (Ed.). (1995). *Neurological Rehabilitation* (3rd ed.). St. Louis, MO: Mosby.

Van Deusen, J., & Brunt, D. (1997). *Assessment in Occupational Therapy and Physical Therapy*. Philadelphia: WB Saunders.

Vance, H. B. (1993). *Best Practices in Assessment for School and Clinical Settings*. Brandon, VT: Clinical Psychology Publishing.

Wallace H., Biehl, R., MacQuenn, J., & Blackman, J. (Eds.). (1997). *Mosby's Resource Guide to Children With Disabilities and Chronic Illness*. St Louis, MO: Mosby.

Whitmore, K., Hart, H., & Willems, G. (Eds.). (1999). *A Neurodevelopmental Approach to Specific Learning Disorders*. London: MacKeith Press.

Widerstrom, A., Mowder, B., & Sandall, S. (1997). *Infant Development and Risk: An Sntroduction* (2nd ed.). Baltimore, MD: Paul H. Brookes.

Wilhelm, I. J., (Ed). (1993). *Physical Therapy Assessment in Early Infancy*. New York, NY: Churchill-Livingstone.

Winter, D. (1990). *Biomechanics and Motor Control of Human Movement* (2nd ed.). New York, NY: John Wiley & Sons.

Wolery, M., & Wilbers, J. (Eds.). (1994). *In-*

cluding Children With Special Needs in Early Childhood Programs. Washington, DC: National Association for the Education of Young Children.

Wolf, L., & Glass, R. (1992). *Feeding and Swallowing Disorders in Infancy: Assessment and Management.* San Antonio, TX: Therapy Skill Builders.

Woolacott, M., & Shumway-Cook, A. (Eds.). (1989). *Development of Posture and Gait Across the Life Span.* Columbia, SC: University of South Carolina Press.

Wyly, M. V. (Ed.). (1995). *Premature Infants and Their Families: Developmental Interventions.* San Diego, CA: Singular.

Ysseldyke, J., & Thurlow, M. (Eds.). (1995). *Educational Outcomes for Students With Disabilities.* Binghamton, NY: Haworth Press.

Zaichkin, J. (1996). *Newborn Intensive Care: What Every Parent Needs to Know.* Petaluma, CA: NICU Book Publishers.

JOURNALS

American Journal of Mental Retardation
American Association of Mental
  Retardation
Washington, DC

American Journal of Occupational Therapy
American Association of Occupational
  Therapy
Bethesda, MD

Archives of Disease in Children
BMJ Publishers Group
London, England

Child Development
Blackwell Publishers
Malden, MA

*Developmental Medicine and Child
  Neurology*
MacKeith Press
London, England

Exceptional Children
Council for Exceptional Children
Reston, VA

Infancy
Lawrence Erlbaum Associates, Publishers
Mahwah, NJ

Infant Behavior and Development
Elsevier Science, Inc.
New York, NY

*Infant and Toddler Intervention:
  The Transdisciplinary Journal*
Singular Publishers
San Diego, CA

Infants and Young Children
Aspen Publishers
Gaithersburg, MD

Journal of Early Intervention
Council for Exceptional Children
Reston, VA

Mental Retardation
American Association of Mental
  Retardation
Washington, DC

*Neonatal Network: The Journal of
  Neonatal Nursing*
Santa Rosa, CA

Pediatric Physical Therapy
Lippincott, Williams & Wilkins
Philadelphia, PA

Physical Therapy
American Physical Therapy Association
Alexandria, VA

*Physical and Occupational Therapy in
  Pediatrics*
Haworth Press
Binghamton, NY

*Topics in Early Childhood Special
  Education*
Pro-ed
Austin, TX

Zero to Three
ZERO to THREE : National Center for
  Infants, Toddlers, and Families
Washington, DC

INDEX

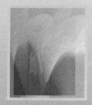

Page numbers in *italics* denote figures; those followed by "t" denote tables or boxes.

285

INDEX